Pregnancy
Mindfulness Technique
for a *Positive* Birthing Experience.

How to Balance your Mind and Your Body for a Natural, Pain-Free and Confident Childbirth.

Anne Mary Holmes

© **Copyright 2020 by Anne-Mary Holmes- All rights reserved.**

This document is geared towards providing exact and reliable information in regard to the topic and issue covered.

- From a Declaration of Principles which was accepted and approved equally by a Committee of the American Bar Association and a Committee of Publishers and Associations.

In no way is it legal to reproduce, duplicate, or transmit any part of this document in either electronic means or in printed format. All rights reserved.

The information provided herein is stated to be truthful and consistent, in that any liability, in terms of inattention or otherwise, by any usage or abuse of any policies, processes, or directions contained within is the solitary and utter responsibility of the recipient reader. Under no circumstances will any legal responsibility or blame be held against the publisher for any reparation, damages, or monetary loss due to the information herein, either directly or indirectly.

Respective authors own all copyrights not held by the publisher.

The information herein is offered for informational purposes solely and is universal as so. The presentation of the information is without contract or any type of guarantee assurance.

The trademarks that are used are without any consent, and the publication of the trademark is without permission or backing by the trademark owner. All trademarks and brands within this book are for clarifying purposes only and are owned by the owners themselves, not affiliated with this document.

Table of Contents

Introduction 7

Chapter 1: How does Your Mind work? 11

Chapter 2: Mindfulness for Birth 19

Chapter 3: The Hypnobirthing Philosophy 27

Chapter 4: The Benefits of a Mindful Hypnobirthing 35

Chapter 5: Getting Ready for a Mindful Hypnobirthing 43

Chapter 6: How to Practice Hypnobirthing 49

Chapter 7: Getting to Know your Birthing zone 55

Chapter 8: Letting Go of Fear and Anxiety 63

Chapter 9: Techniques 71

Chapter 10: Breathing Technique 77

Chapter 11: The Power of Visualization for Birth ... 91

Chapter 12: What is a Birth Plan, and Why is it Important? 97

Chapter 13: When will birth begin? 119

Chapter 14: The Birth 127

Chapter 15: The Umbilical Code 137

Chapter 16: Have a Green and Gorgeous Pregnancy .. 143

Chapter 17: Yoga and Childbirth 153

Chapter 18: Visualization and Childbirth 157

Chapter 19: In Control 165

Chapter 20: Relaxation During Childbirth 173

Chapter 21: Sources of Childbirth Pangs 181

Chapter 21: Post Birth Changes for Mom 189

Chapter 22: Baby Sleep Problems 195

Chapter 23: Breastfeeding Basics: Tips for Successful Feedings 203

Chapter 24: What Do I Need to take in the Hospital? 211

Conclusion 217

The hand that rocks the cradle rules the world.

William Ross Wallace

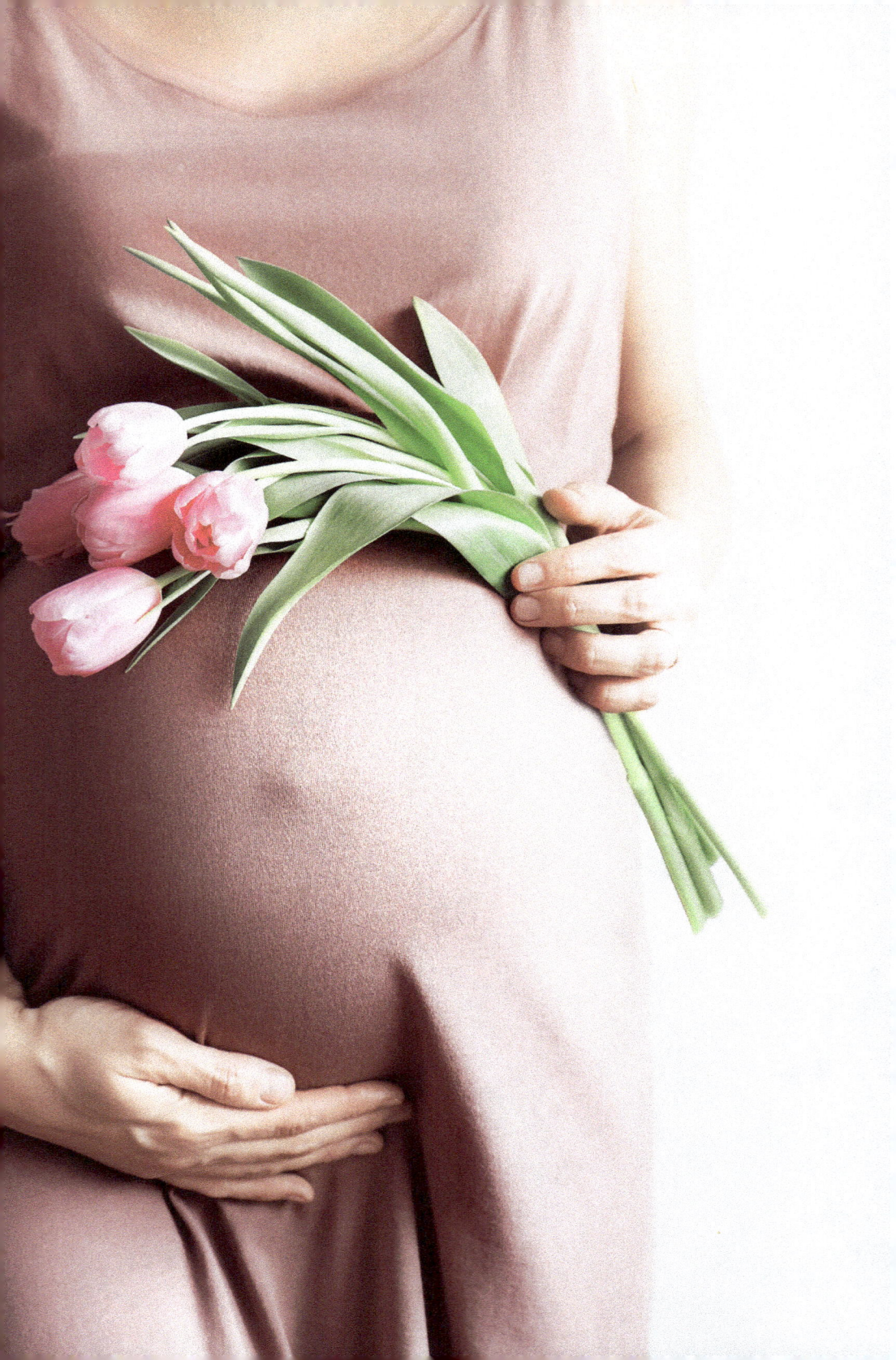

Introduction

Natural Pregnancy and birth are so far from the social norm now because technology, isolation, and unnatural work environments, among other factors, infiltrate all areas of life. Not being in nature, in community, and not quieting the mind to listen to ourselves separates us on all levels.

Humans have evolved as a social species – we require community and support and closeness to others. We are also of nature. Biologically, we have been (and still are) able to reproduce quickly to maintain our species.

If the body could not conceive, carry, and birth a baby naturally, none of us would exist.

So, what happened that so many now mistrust this ability?

Feel it needs to be managed, monitored at the very least? Aside from the lack of connection and trust, our bodies are indeed less prepared for the task. Poor food choices, sitting all day long, and lack of knowledge and support at birth all lower our bodies' capability to function at their best. We are all capable of walking many miles, for example, but how we can fulfill that task can vary significantly from person to person depending on their current activity level, their diet, and their overall health. Birth is natural but not necessarily easy.

Pregnancy comes with a whole hormonal activity upheaval,

changes to organ locations, added weight, increased circulation, and changed metabolism. The demands placed on the body during this period are like those of an athlete that is in training. Their body is also in a state of heightened performance. When resources are allocated to those functions, the immune system is lowered. You can't fight infections as well when you are growing a baby. There have been numerous studies to show that mothers in poor health or those whose immune systems were activated during pregnancy had poorer birth outcomes. They were sicker, and their children were less healthy than those who had mothers in optimal health. During pregnancy, the child always gets what he needs first, given its availability. The mother may be suffering from low vitamin levels, but her fetus will not. It's simple species survival.

This biological programming is acknowledged in mainstream medicine. Somehow, women are advised to increase their vitamin intake, sleep more, and drink more water. But the question is, what about the rest, such as fixing their health and boosting their immune systems? Or their need for exercising in preparation for one of the most taxing physical activities of their lives?

Then add an understanding of their babies. Many women today have never even been around a newborn before they have their own. Before they give birth themselves, they don't hear other birth stories. Unless they have a knowledgeable doula, midwife, or older female family member, chances are they won't know of too many techniques to manage their labor comfortably without taking a class or researching online. A commitment to having a natural birth without all this preparation is like making a wish to run a marathon and preparing for it by reading motivational running books on your couch.

Pregnancy and childbirth are a physical, mental, and emotional journey. The body matures through it and fulfills its task best sequentially. We go through puberty as we move from childhood to adulthood. Moving from a pre-baby form to a post-baby requires us to move through pregnancy. It is not just a task our bodies do, but our minds also need to shift and change into ones caring for this other life. After pregnancy starts, we are no longer a single person. We now think, eat, breathe, and feel for another as well. It is just as important as the physical part. After all, by the time we give birth, we've had quite some time on this earth learning the customs and social requirements of our culture while our baby had none and needs to adjust to this new world. Being able to communicate gently and effectively will ease the transition considerably.

We are all connected through one spirit. Even those who deny it have undoubtedly felt at least once in their life a particular connection to another person. It is as if they've known them before or are reunited with an old friend. Just as we have a soul, so do our children. We have a purpose on this earth, just as they do. Merely understanding should help you see them as their person – one worthy of feelings, respect, preferences, and their journey through life. We not only teach them, but they also teach us.

If we are mentally disconnected, unaware, or fearful, it is hard to be indeed present and care for beings that are still so close to nature when we are so far. It is easy to get angry when the baby is still not sleeping quietly alone all night at one year old, when the toddler dawdles on a walk collecting leaves every few feet, when the newborn fusses whenever you set them down.

We evolved as an intelligent, social, caring species. That

means we need to know others are around for survival. Babies need to be held and nursed; often, we are interested in our surroundings and tune with others' feelings and emotions. A lot of this comes into play after birth when you are caring for your newborn, but it is a lot easier to do if you take the time during pregnancy to address any mental blocks you may have and work through them leading up to the birth.

You will learn how to reconnect your body with nature through food – optimizing your health and supporting your pregnancy. You will learn how to exercise in a way that prepares you for birth while considering any physical limitations you may currently have. You will learn how to address any parenting fears or doubts you may have, any anxieties that keep you from quieting your mind, any concern you may have about the birth itself, and any shortcomings you feel you have and don't want to keep carrying with you. You will acquire how to reinforce your relationship with your partner and your baby so that you can be a united family with shared values and visions. You will discover many tools to birth the way you wish.

Birth is unpredictable, each child's arrival is unique, and the device you were prepared to use may not be the one you need – it's good to have multiple options. You will learn how to choose your birth team and what your options are to support you in having the birth experience you wish. You will know how to hold onto your vision in case things go differently and be able to accept the changes by choice instead of by default. Finally, you will get a good connection to what baby is experiencing as they go through their transition, and through that understanding, you will be able to strengthen your bond in parenting to make the best choices for both of you.

Chapter 1: How does Your Mind work?

Mind, Conscious, and Subconscious

As you're setting goals consciously, if your subconscious mind is not on board with your plans due to what your critical mind judges to be true or false based on your programming, you may be left unable to draw up enough motivation to achieve that goal. Remember: the subconscious mind is responsible for your inspiration and is merely running the programs it knows. For example, you may consciously tell yourself that you want to stop judging other people, however, if you were conditioned to pick out other people's flaws. It might be because that's what your learned was "normal" based on your family dynamic. Your subconscious mind will continue running that program, automatically judging other people, leaving you feeling disappointed in yourself and unable to stop this habit.

So, with that critical mind in the way, how do you communicate with your subconscious mind?

Is there a dream of yours that feels too real, but upon waking up, it made absolutely no sense? When you are dreaming, your subconscious mind is free to play and explore. During sleep, your critical mind has turned off, allowing your subconscious mind to construct nonsensical scenes of its choosing. When you wake up, and your critical mind is back at work, do you consciously think, "Wow, that was a strange dream." It gives us an important clue for how best to communicate with our subconscious minds.

Your subconscious mind can certainly still listen to commands while you are asleep. But I realized that the most effective approach to reprogram yourself is by remaining conscious but putting yourself into a state of deep relaxation. By staying awake, you reduce the risk of your subconscious mind entering that nonsensical dream state.

Being in a state of deep relaxation allows your critical mind to loosen its grip and stop questioning everything that you are suggesting to yourself. You must enable your vital mind to relax, so it does not interfere with the positive changes you want to make.

For example, let us say that you struggle with low self-esteem and want to reprogram yourself for confidence. Imagine that you are giving yourself the suggestion, "You are overflowing with a sense of confidence and can achieve whatever it is that you set out to do." This suggestion sounds very contradictory to your critical mind since you struggle with feelings of low self-esteem. Because again, low self-esteem is the program your subconscious is running and has become truth to your critical mind.

If you are under hypnosis, your critical mind backs off, allowing that positive suggestion about confidence and achievement to enter at the subconscious level. With the crucial reason out of the way, the command to be confident can be accepted by your subconscious mind because your subconscious mind cannot rationalize. Again, it obeys the commands you give it.

Hypnosis and Subconscious

Let us talk about how you can get yourself into a state of relaxation, which will allow your critical mind to back off so you can give positive commands to your subconscious mind. As I mentioned initially, I am a Hypnotherapist, but I made self-hypnosis recordings long before I was certified.

Technically, all hypnosis is self-hypnosis. Even when working with a Hypnotherapist, you are entirely in control and cannot be forced to do anything against your will. Your mind only accepts the suggestions that align with your values and the goals you are trying to achieve. The self-hypnosis I am referring to, however, is in the form of an audio recording that includes relaxation techniques and positive suggestions, as opposed to working with someone in-person.

Type of Language Used to Communicate with Your Subconscious Mind

- **Repetition**

Your subconscious mind needs repetition to form new, positive habits. Therefore, I advised that for this first reprogramming process, you focus on one goal or personal quality that you want to cultivate.

When you communicate with your subconscious mind, you do not necessarily want to say the same statement repeatedly; however, you'll want to create variations of your suggestions that are pointing toward the common goal. You will see variations for proposals related to confidence, and you will learn how long your list of tips should be.

- **Speaking in First vs. Second Person**

Before getting started, you will want to decide if you wish to give your suggestions in the first person, by using the word, I, or in the second person, by using the name, you. Here is the same suggestion for confidence given in the two tenses:

First Person: I wake up each day feeling confident and proud of the person I am.

Second Person: You wake up each day feeling confident and proud of the person you are.

I found that when I first started training my subconscious mind, it felt more comfortable hearing the suggestions in the second person using you. In the beginning, I hadn't quite learned how to relax as deeply as I can now, so I think that my critical mind would have put up some resistance to me saying that I was already confident when I wasn't. Having "someone else," say it, or at least that is how it comes across when you hear the word, you were more believable.

Many of my clients come into my program with inner critic voices that talk to them in the second person, saying things like, "You shouldn't have done that. You must go to the gym. You, you, you" So, writing suggestions in your format helps change how their inner critic speaks to them throughout the day.

Now that my conscious and subconscious minds are in alignment and I can relax very quickly, I write my suggestions in the first person. It is entirely up to you, and there is no right or wrong way about it, but if you are not sure, I recommend starting by writing in the second person. All the following examples will be written in the "you" form.

- **Speaking in Positive Terms**

When you communicate with your subconscious mind, you always want to speak positively and avoid negatives. Speaking in negative terms can cause you to attract what you do not wish to. For example, if I said to you, "Don't think about a giant yellow snake with red bunny ears," what are you most likely to think about?

However, not everything that we want to achieve in terms of personal development is positive, right? In addition to creating more positive thoughts, feelings, and habits, there are specific thoughts, feelings, and traditions we no longer want to have. Luckily, creative ways of wording these types of suggestions so they do not involve negative words like "can't, don't, won't, no, no."

For example, let us say you are programming yourself for confidence. You want to include positive suggestions for confidence, self-esteem, and optimism. Besides, a great way to increase trust is to stop worrying about what other people think about you.

Here is a "negative" way of putting that suggestion, which we want to avoid:

One should not be concerned about what other people think of them.

Because your subconscious mind doesn't process negatives

well, that suggestion could be interpreted as, "You worry about what other people think about you," which is the exact opposite of what you are trying to achieve!

Here are a few creative ways that you could modify the suggestion to have the right effect:

•   You have stopped worrying about what others think about you.

•   You let go of worrying about what others think of you.

•   You interact easily with others without worrying about what they are thinking of you.

There is an exception to the rule when it comes to using negative terms. Let us say that you have a powerful suggestion that uses a negative time. In that case, you want to follow up that statement with a positive alternative immediately. In other words, if you are telling your subconscious not to do something, what do you want it to do instead?

Here is an example:

What other people think about you no longer even crosses your mind.

The "no" in this statement makes this a negative suggestion. It could be interpreted as the opposite of what you intended. You would want to follow up that suggestion with a positive statement, telling your subconscious mind what to do instead, like so:

What other people think about you no longer even crosses your mind.

Instead, you always assume that others feel the best of you, so you let go of worrying that they are judging you.

I do not want you to worry too much about scrutinizing your suggestions. Just be mindful that when you are using negative terms and look for creative ways to reword the requests so that your subconscious mind can be more receptive to them.

- **Speaking in Present Tense and Visualizing Your Goal Has Come True**

The quickest way to bring about the positive changes you want to see is to speak to your subconscious mind as if you have already achieved your goal. It is the same reason why visualizing your success as if it has already happened is a more effective strategy than imagining that success will happen sometime in the vague future.

What's more powerful for your imagination: telling yourself that someday you'll own that villa in Greece, or imagining the estate is yours right now, seeing yourself walking around the house, hanging out with all of your friends, and knowing that if you have that villa right now, you must have reached your wealth goals and all of the positive things that entail?

Considering this is one of the daily goals I imagine, I can tell you with certainty that the second scenario is MUCH more powerful. Imagining that I already have the villa in Greece gets me so excited that I continue pressing forward in my business to make that a reality as soon as possible. If I imagined that it would happen someday, there is an air of uncertainty, making it much less potent in my mind.

You always want to use the present tense when you are programming yourself for personal qualities as well. For example, instead of saying, "You are going to be confident," which is a vague way of creating confidence because it has no tangible timeframe of when that confidence is going to come about, you would want to say it in the present tense like so:

You are overflowing with an abundance of self-confidence, self-love, and self-esteem.

Your confidence pours out of you so strongly that everyone around you takes notice.

Can you imagine what things you would be doing knowing that you are already overflowing with self-confidence, self-love, and self-esteem? Can you visualize the people around you noticing your confidence and how amazing that feels?

Chapter 2: Mindfulness for Birth

Our minds control our emotions, our bodies, and our behavior. When we train our minds, we increase our power to help achieve our goals and desires. What specifically are your dreams and desires right now?

- Do you want to experience a joyful, fulfilling pregnancy?
- Do you wish to achieve a superior birthing performance that is natural, safe, pain-free, and comfortable?
- Do you want a normal, healthy, and happy baby?
- Can you see yourself achieving these goals?
- Are you willing to commit the time and effort needed to prepare yourself to achieve these goals?
- Do these goals excite you and move you to action?

Answering "yes" to these questions puts you on the path to success; so, let us begin.

Your mental training will cover the following areas:
1. Improving your concentration and focus of attention
2. Monitoring and managing your thoughts
3. Developing and utilizing imaging and creative visualization skills
4. They are learning self-hypnosis and Hypno-meditation.

The mental skills outlined above will enable you to attain a state of mind which blocks the negative thoughts and physical discomfort that interfere with your focus on the birthing process and your enjoyment of this experience.

First, let me remind you of the unlimited power of that fantastic bio-computer, the brain. You have two sides of your mind: the left and the right hemispheres. The left brain is dominant in logic, words, numbers, sequence, analysis, lists, and linearity. The right mind is dominant in rhythm, imagination, intuition, daydreaming, color, gestalt (whole picture), and spatial awareness. In our civilized world, greater emphasis and importance is placed on the development of left-brain skills. Thus, leaving right-brain gifts underdeveloped and underutilized. Tony Buzan, in his book, Use Your Head, tells us that by stimulating and utilizing the skills of both sides of the brain, we can learn to do anything and do it with excellence.

Pregnancy and birthing are essentially multi-sensory, holistic experiences involving every aspect of our total being—physical, mental, emotional, and spiritual. The brain controls the functioning of all these areas. We, therefore, need the integrated use of the cognitive skills of both sides of the brain to enable us better to develop these capabilities and to achieve our goals.

All the exercises are designed to develop the mental skills of both sides of your brain so that you can utilize "whole-brain" functioning. Mental gymnastics is just as important as physical exercise. It will strengthen your power during pregnancy and birthing and in all other areas of your life.

1. Improving Your Concentration and Focus of Attention

The success of any of our endeavors is determined essentially by our ability. It is to maintain a focus of attention on the task at hand. It requires a high level of mental discipline. A mother-to-be will be necessary to focus her attention on the specific task of birthing her baby and not be disturbed by personal discomfort or external distractions. Here are two exercises that will help you to strengthen this ability.

EXERCISE 1: Focusing Your Attention

You can begin by only focusing your attention on a flower. Keep your eyes glued to the flower of your choice. Hold it about 18 inches away from you and allow yourself to observe it closely. Notice the texture, size, shape, and color of its petals. Look deeply at its center. Then contemplate its nature. Afterward, spend 5-10 minutes in focused attention. If your attention strays when an extraneous thought enters your mind, just let it go and bring your attention gently back to the flower. You can practice this exercise with any small object. You may use a ball, a fruit, or a pen, or the flame of a lighted candle. Perform this exercise at least once a day or as often as you can. As you increase your power of concentration, you will find that it becomes easier for you to relax any part of your body at will and maintain an inner calm.

EXERCISE 2: Brain Fitness Exercise

It is a beneficial exercise for improving your overall brain performance. It will also give you greater control of your thoughts, improve your mental alertness, memory, and increase your peripheral vision and speed-reading ability.

- Sit on a chair with your back straight and your feet flat on the floor. Allow your hands to rest unclasped on your lap

- Focus on a small spot at a 45-degree angle. Keep your eyes glued to that spot. You may blink if necessary but try not to shift your eyes.

Identify:
- Three things you see
- Three things you hear
- Three things you feel

Find:
- Two new things you see
- Two new things you hear
- Two new things you feel

Pinpoint:
- One unique thing you see
- One unique thing you hear
- One unique something you feel

- Close your eyes and breathe slowly and deeply three times

- Say with conviction:

"I control my thoughts.

I control my feelings.

I control my actions.

And God is helping me in every way."

- Open your eyes, take a deep breath, and stretch.

This exercise is based on the Betty Erickson Technique for self-hypnosis. You will find that it can also help you to go more quickly and deeply into self-hypnosis or meditation since it prevents wandering thoughts and allows you to focus your mind.

I remember doing an exercise like this one (without the breathing, affirmations, and spiritual component) when I first went back to university to do my master's in counseling psychology. I was the oldest student in the class, and I felt I had cobwebs on my brain. The other younger students were so quick and alert! I needed to activate my mind functioning to enable me to concentrate for more extended periods and to memorize and recall faster and more accurately. I discovered this concentration exercise, and it was suggested that I do it once or twice a day. I added the affirmations, and I was so motivated that I practiced it 4-5 times a day! I placed post-its stickers all over the house to remind me to do it. I practiced in the bathroom, and while watching TV (during advertisements), I practiced it on the patio, in the car (before starting to drive), and at my study desk; I practiced it while sitting, standing, or lying in bed. It was a great way to refresh myself, clear my head, or help me to fall asleep. The good news is that it worked for me.

And it can do for you too!

Monitoring and Managing Your Thoughts

"A man is what he thinks all day long."

Ralph Waldo Emerson

There is a constant interaction between your thoughts, your feelings, and your actions.

For example: (a) If you think that someone is coming to harm you, you will feel fear and hostility towards them, and then. As a result, you may have to choose aggressive or defensive action. (fight or take flight):

THOUGHTS→FEELINGS→ACTIONS

(b) If you are doing charitable work (step), you can increase your empathy for others (feeling) and strengthen the belief (thought) that we need to help each other.

ACTION→FEELINGS→THOUGHTS

(c) If you feel anger towards someone, you will probably think negative thoughts about that person, which can trigger a defensive or aggressive reaction.

FEELINGS→THOUGHTS→ACTIONS

So, we need to manage our thoughts, our feelings, and our actions. Let us now focus on managing the quality of our reviews, which can be the most difficult to control. Scientific research has shown that the quality of our thoughts affects the chemistry in our bodies.

Negative thoughts change the frequency of the neurotransmitters in the brain and give rise to chemicals such as cortisol and adrenaline that affects our bodily functions and can lead to aggressive or depressed behavior. These negative thoughts become limiting paradigms and prevent us from developing our fullest potential and enjoying the fullness of life.

Positive thoughts also affect the frequency of the neurotransmitters in the brain, which secrete other chemicals such as oxytocin and endorphins that lift the spirit, energize the body, and produce positive behavior. So obviously, we must learn to think more positive thoughts. That is easier said than done, but with the effort, it can be done. There are several ways of managing ideas that flow through our minds. The key to this is to get into the habit of being sufficiently aware of our thoughts to monitor them continuously. The positive ones we can foster. The negatives ones we can cancel out and replace with more positive ones. Begin with these two practical exercises.

EXERCISE 1: Cancelling Negative Thoughts

Let us look at some negative thoughts, general ones, and those specific to pregnancy and birthing.

1.List your negative thoughts in the left-hand column of the following table.

2.Cancel out each of these negative thoughts, saying to yourself emphatically "Cancel that!" and putting an X over all the negatives.

3.Transform each negative thought into a complimentary, empowering view and write it in the column on the right. Here are some guidelines for creating empowering beliefs:

- Keep it simple.
- Keep it short.
- Keep it positive.
- Keep it in the present tense.
- Use these positive thoughts as affirmations.

It is how it goes: "Birthing will be painful." (negative thought) Say firmly, "Cancel that!" or "Delete! Delete!" Then affirm: "Birthing is comfortable and natural."

I have given you some examples of how you can transform these negatives thoughts into empowering thoughts. Complete the transformation of any other negative thoughts that you may have on your list.

Chapter 3: The Hypnobirthing Philosophy

What is Mindful Hypnobirthing?

Hypnobirthing is an approach to managing pain, as well as stress and anxiety, throughout childbirth. It includes various therapeutic relaxation techniques, such as deep breathing and visualization.

It's essentially taking those old beliefs and thoughts around childbirth, which were triggering anxiety, and then transforming those old beliefs to new ones that will positively equip you for delivery. Hypnobirthing then includes adding functional healing techniques and teaching you to change your attitude to give you the excellent birthing experience that you prefer.

It is a birthing strategy that consolidates extensive breathing, unwinding, representation, self-mesmerizing, and direction for both you and your birthing partner. You can use the systems in labor as well as transportation to aid you in adapting to pain.

An Example

Testimon of Kristine F:

«My second daughter was an induction. She was showing as over nine pounds on the ultrasound measurements, and I was built tiny. My first baby was eight pounds even, and they were scared that I wouldn't be able to have a baby that was over eight pounds, much less over nine, so they were inducing me to make sure my "little" Annabelle didn't grow any bigger before she made her appearance.

I was induced with my first child, a beautiful little girl, and I knew how horrible inductions were. I had heard how wonderful hypnobirthing was and how much of a difference it made, so I decided to give it a try.

For my visualization, I chose a beautiful waterfall in the middle of the jungle. I pictured myself standing on a large, flat rock beside the bubbling river at the base of the falling water. I have a great imagination, so it was easy for me to get into the visualization—so much so that I could feel the water hit my face and smell the water droplets in the air. I would watch as a beautiful yellow butterfly with black-tipped wings flew in front of me, between me and the waterfall. I would follow it with my eyes as it crossed in front of the falls and into the jungle. Before it would reach the wilderness, I would be through my contraction, and I would start over with the next one.

Did it get boring visualizing the same thing over and over? No. It was comforting. It was beautiful. It was my special place. It was familiar to me. I had created it. I could control it. It seemed to be the only thing I could handle at the time, which made it the perfect place to retreat to during a contraction.

I made it through the delivery with hypnobirthing. Annabelle was ten pounds and eight ounces! As soon as I pushed her out, the nurse assisting the OB exclaimed, "Oh my God!"

I thought there was something wrong with my baby. Nope. I had just birthed a toddler. I hadn't had any difficulty, either. She was out within eighteen minutes of pushing labor. The doctor credited it all to my ability to relax throughout the process. And the only reason I was able to relax was because of the hypnobirthing method. »

How Does Hypnobirthing Work?

Hypnobirthing makes use of individual systems to transfer your concentration away from the fear, uneasiness, and pain that are regularly associated with labor--who hasn't heard countless gloomy birth tales? These methods ready you for birth, assist you with really feeling peaceful, and sure and engage you to feel in charge of the delivery of your baby.

What Techniques and Methods Are Utilized During Hypnobirthing?

Regulated Breathing Activities

If you concentrate on taking long, deep breaths in through your nose and out through your mouth, it encourages you to remain peaceful and maintains your mind's focus.

Understanding

Awareness techniques aid you to envision or 'dream' concerning the introduction of your baby. Including how it will certainly feel and how it will progress. It is done with the goal that you can make a positive experience in your mind that you can go back to. It will also allow you to practice the technique repeatedly before you go into labor.

Extensive Relaxing and Representation

You'll practice the techniques to aid you with shutting out outside confusion so you can concentrate specifically on your body and the well-being of your new baby as you bring him or her into the world.

Favorable Language

Hypnobirthing takes on an alternative approach to speaking as well as taking into consideration the birth experience to decrease fear as well as negativity. For example, contractions are alluded to as 'waves' or 'impressions' that have direction.

Hypnobirthing systems can be used in early labor as well as later during hard labor and delivery. You can make use of the courses in blend with various other things, such as music and positive thinking, with your visualization and hypnosis experience and with different types of remedy for pain. Hypnobirthing isn't just for natural childbirth—the system can also be effectively utilized if things don't go precisely by a plan by aiding you in resisting panic and remaining focused on bringing that precious baby into the world.

Does Hypnobirthing Work?

There is no straightforward answer to this question, as there are only a few studies that have evaluated its use. While a few ladies depend on it enabled them to have a lively labor and delivery experience due to the lowered need for pain medication, other women in the study didn't feel altered anything for them.

The idea of hypnobirthing, however, is becoming more widespread and well-liked. Aided by maternity specialists, a couple of NHSs (National Health Services) in the UK are currently supplying hypnobirthing as routine pain management.

My husband and I both made use of hypnobirthing with our very first baby. Also, it was a Godsend when I was having withdrawals from cigarettes, as it helped me to relax, regulate my breathing, take control of my mind, and get through it.

What Makes It So Great?

There are a couple of reasons that the pain drug alternative, hypnobirthing, might intrigue you:

- The steps taken in hypnobirthing can ready your body

and mind for when hard labor starts and encourage you to feel accountable and engaged throughout the birthing of your infant.

- If you or your baby have had hard or devastating labor or delivery, understanding the approach of hypnobirthing before engaging in the struggle may assist you with feeling overwhelmed by your feelings of fear, sadness, or devastation.

- You might need much less added aid with discomfort, despite the reality that hypnobirthing can be utilized with other relief from discomfort choices on the occasion that you choose.

- You can use hypnobirthing in the hospital, a birthing center, or during a home birth. It can be used with any kind of birth plan very quickly.

- The great news is that you can take your birthing partner along to the hypnobirthing programs (classes during pregnancy) with you. This exercise can better them at their job on the big day.

How Does It Work?

Don't worry, ladies. No one is going to swing a watch in your face. Not until your eyes are spinning in circles, and you're barking like a dog and chasing your tail. You don't even have to go to a classroom to learn hypnobirthing. I didn't. Yes, you can do a private or group class, but you can also do an online course.

The foundation of hypnobirthing is learning to calm your emotions. And who doesn't need to know to control their emotions?

The programs will use several different strategies to show you the exact steps to relax. The reason for all these strategies is twofold: (1) different methods work for other people, and (2) different situations may necessitate a different approach.

A few of the strategies are:

- Knead techniques
- Envisioning
- Breathing strategies
- Perusing or tuning into a reflective chronicle
- And others

The other part of hypnobirthing facilities the birthing process itself. The main principle of hypnobirthing is that being fearful throughout the birthing process can several problems, including delayed labor. So, one thing the classes attempt to is to confront these feelings of dread head-on by battling them with information. Those sayings "information is power" and "fear of the unknown" become possibly one of the essential variables in hypnobirthing.

We understand that we frequently fear the unknown, and labor is among those that continue to be among the most cloudy and obscure. New mothers often feel unsuited to tell other women about their birth experience, so what continues throughout birth is kept quiet. Add to that the details we do have (i.e., movies and reality Television shows) are typical scenes of young girls screaming in pain and dread, encompassed by so many people, nurses, and doctors that they undoubtedly feel suffocated. It should not be a big shock to us that so many women today dread labor.

It is where these hypnotherapy programs come in. They will undoubtedly show women precisely how the body tries to birth a baby, expelling the fear of the unknown, for it is no longer anonymous. Their perspective and belief about birth will then wholly change. They will then testify that labor and delivery do not need to be the frightening experience that so many say that it is. However, fearing it creates virtually the extra pain due to the tension and strains the added anxiety adds upon the body. Both experiences, whether positive or negative, truly become transformative encounters.

I can honestly tell you that I loved carrying each of my children when I found I was pregnant. It is an experience that still, after so many years, always brings a smile to my face—

I owe a ton of that motivation to hypnobirthing.

Chapter 4: The Benefits of a Mindful Hypnobirthing

For a first-time mother, childbirth is the most fearsome and most significant pregnancy-related anxiety that a woman generally faces. It is due to mental pressure, excruciating pain, and various complications they usually undergo. But natural childbirth is an unmediated birth and has lots of hidden benefits. In our society, giving pain medication for labor is so obvious and common that almost all women hanker after that. Doctors assume that most women want it to reduce their pain. But this pain medication has some side effects and can be a cause of adverse circumstances. Almost all women become terrified due to severe pain and wish for getting an epidural. But you shouldn't forget that epidural is a drug, and most drugs have some side effects.

There is another side of this story and a possible solution for this drug-free labor: natural childbirth with the assistance of midwives. The advantages of natural childbirth are many, and some women still opt to give birth naturally.

Benefits of Natural Childbirth

There are quite a few benefits that natural childbirth can provide to a woman.

1. Emotional and psychological advantages - Birthing children naturally is a courageous task on account of a woman, and for that, you need strength, courage, and support always. The woman who delivers naturally feels an empowering experience, and only she can feel how strong, powerful, and prepared she is both emotionally and psychologically. Researchers point out that a newborn and its mother on pain medication during birth may face trouble bonding right away. And this is stressful for mothers. But the emotional and psychological relationship is established immediately in respect of natural breeding.

2. Speedy and faster childbirth - The next significant advantage is that natural breeding is quicker and safer. Pushing helps the baby come out faster, and in natural birth, a mother can feel the intensity of whether she is pushing harder or not. But the use of anesthesia, such as an epidural, prevents her from feeling that sense of passion. Besides, the effectiveness of contractions and labor isn't slowed down in this natural process. The more the mother can push, the faster the baby comes out.

3. Benefits of skipping medication and pain relief - The use of epidural and other medications during childbirth dramatically affects the health of the mother and her child. All these drugs can help you reduce the pain, but they have side effects like nausea, vomiting, drowsiness, dizziness, confusion, and more. Also, all drugs used during the childbirth cross the placenta and significantly affect and damage your baby's health. Besides, epidurals have side effects such as significant blood pressure drops, fever, and detachment from reality, itchy feeling, lumbar puncture, and spinal headache. A newborn can be groggy, tired, and sleepy for using medications. But natural childbirth shuns the damage or side effects of drugs and drugs and helps smooth the growth of the baby and ensures sound health and brain.

4.Breastfeeding is more comfortable and smoother - In natural childbirth, breastfeeding seems more relaxed, natural, and softer than who received pain medications and epidurals. The babies born through natural breeding are more alert and show more interest in breastfeeding once delivered. The woman who receives pain medications and epidurals, suffers from the senselessness and drugged, and it passes to her babies as well. Pain medications can hinder the babies' natural and innate suckling power and strength. But in natural birth, a woman feels no hindrance in breastfeeding, and babies are spontaneous in that act.

5.Labor and contraction are often faster and shorter - Pain-relieving medications and epidurals often slow down the labor process and create impediments in natural contractions. These medications often lead to slower delivery. Besides, women generally do not feel their contractions and do not know when to push. On the contrary, natural childbirth facilitates the labor process and enables smooth delivery.

6.Natural childbirth is sound for mom and baby and ensures faster recovery- As no medication and epidural are used in natural birth, it is often healthier for mom and baby. Besides, mom and baby do not feel drugged, and faster recovery is ensured naturally.

7.Natural childbirth is empowering and facilitates better connection- Very often, the woman who goes through the natural birthing process feels incredibly empowered and confident. This spontaneous experience and knowledge also help her in the future to face any obstacle very smoothly. Besides, this process hastens a better connection or relationship between the mother and her child. As drugs are not used during the process, women often seem very alert and conscious all the time. We must not forget that a woman and her child are connected profoundly. But using drugs and epidurals segregate them from that connection.

8.Free movement during labor- In hospitals, during labor, free training is not allowed at all. When birth begins with induction, moms are required to stay in bed during their labor and delivery. Most hospitals use common positions like lithotomic and C-position, which restrict the pelvic outlet and put unnecessary pressure on the perineum. But labor begins spontaneously and naturally in natural childbirth. Women can feel free and select their positions according to their whims. Massage, meditation, water therapy, breathing techniques, positioning, moaning, and hypnosis are commonly used in natural childbirth.

9.Easy Steps to Sound Pregnancy

Natural childbirth is for those who wish for natural, without-pain management interventions and vaginal delivery. A natural and unmediated vaginal birth is achievable and reasonable for pregnant women, and it is safer and faster than the epidural and pain management interventions of childbirth. If you are going through the natural one, these easy steps or tips are for you.

- Have a sound and solid prenatal and postnatal education: You should have solid prenatal and postnatal knowledge and education regarding natural childbirth. Get acquainted with labor and birth work, natural pain management techniques, natural childbirth techniques, breathing, self-hypnosis, relaxation, and other fundamental things to cope with the situation. You must have sound knowledge regarding the postnatal situation also.

Find out the birthing position that seems comfortable for you.

- Seek an experienced doula or health care provider: Pick an experienced and skilled midwife to assist you during the process to hasten and become smooth. Get ready, a doula that has sound experience in midwifery.

- Prepare yourself physically and mentally: Physical and mental preparation and sound planning help a lot in natural childbirth. You shouldn't break down while in labor because it will create a hindrance for your precious one to come out.

- Get your weight balanced: It is highly recommended that you must get your weight balanced. Overweight women feel complications while laboring, and they may need medical interventions. Labor seems smoother to women who aren't bulky, and they face fewer difficulties.

- Find a pleasant atmosphere: The environment plays a vital role in natural childbirth. So, you must select a friendly atmosphere for your delivery. It will be best if fewer people happen to be there.

- Use water as much as possible: For easing pain and relaxation, you can use as much water as you like because water helps remarkably. A shower, bathtub, or birthing pool may help in this regard.

- Learn various coping techniques and labor positioning:

You must cope with the whole situation. So, don't get nervous and courageously face everything. Learn about multiple positioning during labor and select one that is best for you.

- Try harder to push when needed: Pushing helps push out the baby from the mother's womb. Pushing would be easier if you don't lose your consciousness. Try to focus and be alert always. Try to push harder when it is needed.

- Get support from your partner and friends: A supportive practitioner, partner, or friends can lessen your pain by providing mental support and courage. Talk to your partner to regain your strength because labor and delivery is an emotionally and physically draining process.

- Eat a proper meal: Before going through the process, eat a decent meal, and don't starve yourself. Laboring and pushing need much strength, and well-balanced food can help you immensely.

- Breathing exercises and visualization: Don't forget to breathe normally and keep your visualization as straightforward as possible.

Natural Childbirth Techniques

There are several techniques that can be used while trying to labor without any medical interventions in natural childbirth. The different methods used in natural birth are quite famous and have been successfully used for years. If you prefer natural delivery, you can have a glimpse and opt for the right one for you.

Lamaze technique: It is a widely used childbirth technique, and it is a natural and healthy process. This method uses distraction during labor and contractions to lessen the sensation of pain and discomfort. In this method, you will learn controlled deep breathing, massage, concentration, and how to cope with the whole process.

Alexander technique: It is a method that expatiates over ease, balance, freedom of movement, coordination, and flexibility. It is an educative process, and the more you practice, the more you will benefit. It is a technique for sitting, standing, and moving with safety, ease, and efficiency.

Bradley method: This is a natural method which assists women to deliver naturally with few medicines or no medicine at all. It emphasizes on nutrition, exercise, relaxation techniques to balance pain and supportive involvement of the husband and wife.

Water delivery: Water helps immensely during natural childbirth. For relaxation and lessening birth pain, a warm tub of water is used to give birth to a child. Experts believe that it helps babies to enter less light and a good atmosphere. But it is not recommended for high-risk pregnant women.

Hypnosis: The use of hypnosis at the time of labor assists a woman to relax completely, and it is one of the popular techniques used in natural childbirth. The body's muscles can function correctly in a calm, daydream-like atmosphere, but, of course, in a controlled way.

Chapter 5: Getting Ready for a Mindful Hypnobirthing

Getting the Uterus Ready for the Birth

1. Eat fresh pineapple regularly. I suggest you eat these three to four times a week. It is an acid food and may upset your digestive system if you overeat it.

2. Take a raspberry leaf. It can be taken as a tea or, as it is an acquired taste, it can be taken in tablet or liquid form also. Put 15 to 20 drops of the liquid (depending on the make) in a little water and drink.

Start with one cup of tea a day, one tablet or 15 drops in water, and build up gradually to a maximum of four cups of tea, tablets, or sets of drops daily. The tea can be sipped freely during labor too. In my opinion, the liquid method is the best way to ensure you get the correct standard dosage and it is also easily absorbed into the body. Raspberry leaf in all the forms described can be bought from a health shop.

Both pineapple and raspberry leaf contain a uterine tonic and so help to prepare the uterine muscles for the birth.

Eating large amounts of this fruit stimulates the gut and bowel, and because they are the same type of muscle as the uterus, this may cause contractions to start. That is why it is important not to overeat of it unless you want the birth to begin.

Raspberry leaf contains a nourishing source of vitamins (A, B-complex, C and E), minerals (calcium, iron, magnesium, manganese, and phosphorous) and fragrance, an alkaloid, which gives tone to the muscles of the pelvic region and the uterus itself. The vitamins and minerals help your immune system to be stronger and facilitate healthy skin and bone development for the baby. The calcium is necessary for controlling nerve response during childbirth. The fragrance allows the uterus to contract more powerfully and effectively during labor. If you drink the tea during birth, this will help maintain strong contractions, so your baby is born more quickly. It allows the uterus to let go and function as it is designed to.

The high vitamin and mineral content help to replace those that are lost via blood loss in delivery and the alkaloids that are present will also aid in toning the uterus after birth, allowing it to return to its usual size more quickly. It, in turn, means that blood loss after the delivery is minimized.

Breastfeeding Tips

1. To get the nipples in peak condition, if you can, when you are at home, do not wear a bra. If this is too uncomfortable, then get an old bra and cut holes for your nipples. The friction of the nipples on your clothes toughens the nipples, ready for breastfeeding.

2. Use a nipple cream just before birth to keep the nipples

supple. In this way, the nipples do not dry out so quickly due to the suckling of the baby.

There is usually no medical reason why a mother should not feed her child for as long as they want. Breastfeeding is a personal decision, and it is up to the mother to decide what is best for her. However, it has been shown that breastfeeding for even just a few days is beneficial to the baby. I give the reasons for this below.

The initial milk, known as colostrum, is produced for the first three days and contains protein (four times as much as ordinary milk), lactose, vitamins, white blood cells, serum, and protective antibodies. Although it has a yellow color, there is little or no fat present. It also contains a natural laxative to rid the gut of the meconium, which filled the digestive system of the baby when it was in the uterus. This natural laxative is not found in the powdered milk available, nor are the white blood cells and antibodies, which boost the baby's immune system.

Regular breast milk is a waterier suspension containing fats, proteins, mineral salts (main calcium for healthy bone development), and lactose. The powdered kinds of milk simulate this milk. Production of milk continues if the mother breastfeeds.

Perineal Massage

The perineum is the area around the vagina between the vagina and anus. Massaging the perineum, it gradually softens and stretches the vagina and perineal tissue in preparation for the birth. It is especially useful for first-time mothers and women over 30.

Doing this massage will familiarize you with the feeling of the pressure and stretching of the perineum that you will feel when your baby's head is being born. Being aware of these feelings helps you to relax during birth and to participate in your baby's birth actively.

Either you or your partner can do this massage. Use a mirror the first few times and look at the perineum to see what you are doing. It is advisable to massage after a bath, to begin with, softening the surrounding tissues. Make sure you have emptied your bladder and wash your hands before you start. Find a comfortable position that works best for you. Several positions can be used. These are semi-sitting, reclining, squatting against a wall, or standing with one foot raised and resting on the bath, toilet, or chair.

The massage should be done three to four times a week for about four minutes, beginning six weeks before your due date.

By doing this massage, you get the vagina and perineum used to the 'feelings' of the baby being born, and so they stretch more efficiently, as you are much more relaxed at the birth. Many women who have done this massage regularly have found that they did not tear at the birth. Thus, I would recommend that you do this.

Pregnancy Yoga

It is very beneficial at all stages of the pregnancy. It teaches you relaxation through exercise and breathing. It works well with the hypnosis because it reinforces that you can be in control, to deal with the contractions and the birth process.

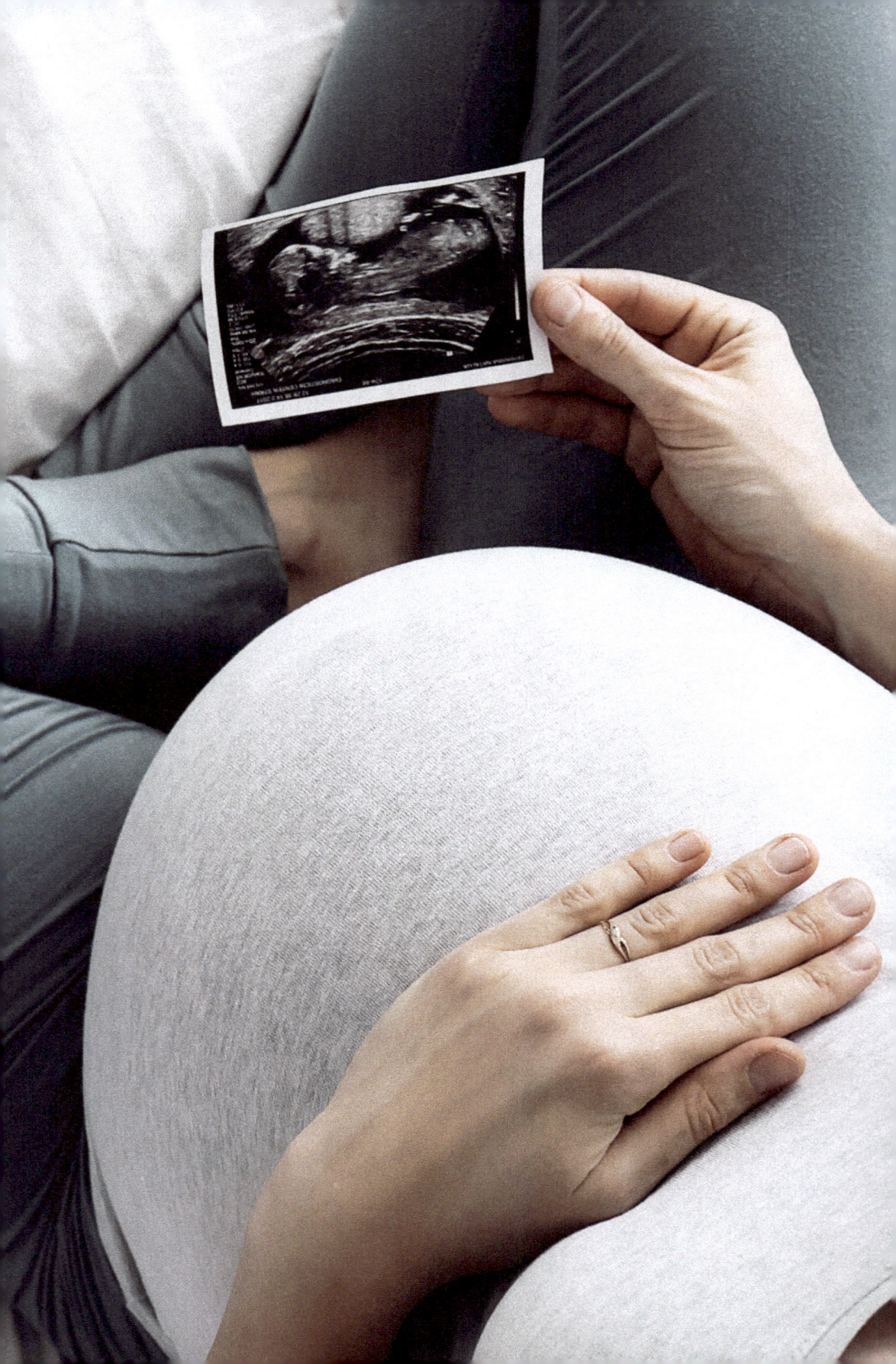

Chapter 6: How to Practice Hypnobirthing

Read A Simple Guidebook to Hypnobirthing

Take your time with it, and as you read, the information will filter down into your unconscious mind. The more you read, the more you understand. The more you know and practice, the more prepared your mind and body will be for a calm and confident birth!

Calming Breath Technique

The Calming Breath can fit into your daily routine, and perhaps you could spend a few minutes practicing before you get out of bed in the morning to calm before you start the day. Or you could practice while resting during the day and when you go to bed so that you prepare yourself for a good night's sleep.

Birthing Breath Technique

The Birthing Breath. This breath should be practiced from week 36.

Positive Thoughts and Words

Remember that what you tell yourself, what you listen to, and read affects how you feel right down to a cellular level. So, keep your thoughts and words positive.

Self-Hypnosis MP3

The right Mp3 playlist can be used to help you feel calm and relaxed.

It will prepare your mind and body for the birth of your baby. You may also listen to this recording at least once a week during pregnancy to help prepare your mind and body for labor. Nearer your Window of Birth, you may wish to listen to the recording at least three times weekly. It is ideal for playing your playlist recording while you are giving birth.

The MP3 will help you to feel more comfortable during pregnancy, the three stages of labor, and reduce the need for pain relief..

Positive Affirmations

It can be used with the Calming Breath and self-hypnosis. You can also write them on post-it notes and place them where you will see them regularly.

Your Color of Comfort and Peace

It can be used to bring calmness and comfort whenever you need it. You may wish to start with The Calming Breath and visualize your color or have an item to hand that reminds you of your chosen color.

Pelvic Floor Exercises

Firstly, let's practice finding your pelvic floor muscles. Make sure that you are sitting, lying, or standing comfortably.

Now squeeze the muscles around the back passage and suppose that you are trying to stop yourself from hitting the wind. Pinch and relax. The legs and buttocks should not move, but you should feel the muscle of the back passage pulling and tightening.

Now envision trying to stop yourself passing on urine. If you are sitting on the toilet, do not stop yourself from passing urine as this can, if continually repeated, cause problems with correct emptying.

There you go! You have hopefully isolated your pelvic floor muscles, remembering the rules of not tightening your buttocks, excessively pulling in your tummy, holding your breath, or squeezing your legs together.

Practicing Pelvic Floor Exercises.

- Stand, lie down or sit with your knees slightly apart. If you are on the toilet, empty your bladder.
- Slowly, draw up the pelvic floor muscles, back passage, front passage, and vagina.
- Lift and squeeze.
- Aim to hold for 10 seconds.
- Relax and rest for 10 seconds.
- Repeat 5-10 times.
- Do this exercise 1-2 times daily.

How to do Perineal Massage

- Choose a time and place where you can relax and won't

be interrupted.

- You can use the Calming Breath to help you feel more relaxed.

- If you cannot reach your perineum easily, then your partner can do it for you using their index fingers instead of their thumbs.

- Choose an unscented oil such as sunflower oil, coconut oil, vitamin E oil, or olive oil.

- Ensure you have washed your hands and that your fingernails are short.

- You may like to have a mirror to hand so you can see what you are doing.

- Find a comfortable position. You can sit, lie down, or stand with one foot on a chair if this is easier for you. Or you can lie in the bath with one foot at a time on the rim.

- Massage some oil on your fingers, thumbs, perineum, and entrance to the vagina.

- Place your thumbs between 2-4cm into your vagina towards the anus and press downwards then outwards, gently pulling your thumbs apart. Hold for a minute or so.

- This way, the perineum is being stretched both downwards and outwards. You may feel a tingling sensation as the perineum stretches.

- Then in a semi-circular motion, starting from the bottom, then moving your thumbs upwards and outwards, and back again, gently massage the area for a few minutes.

Practice one or two times weekly.

*Perineal massage should not hurt. However, if you have any concerns, then please contact your healthcare provider.

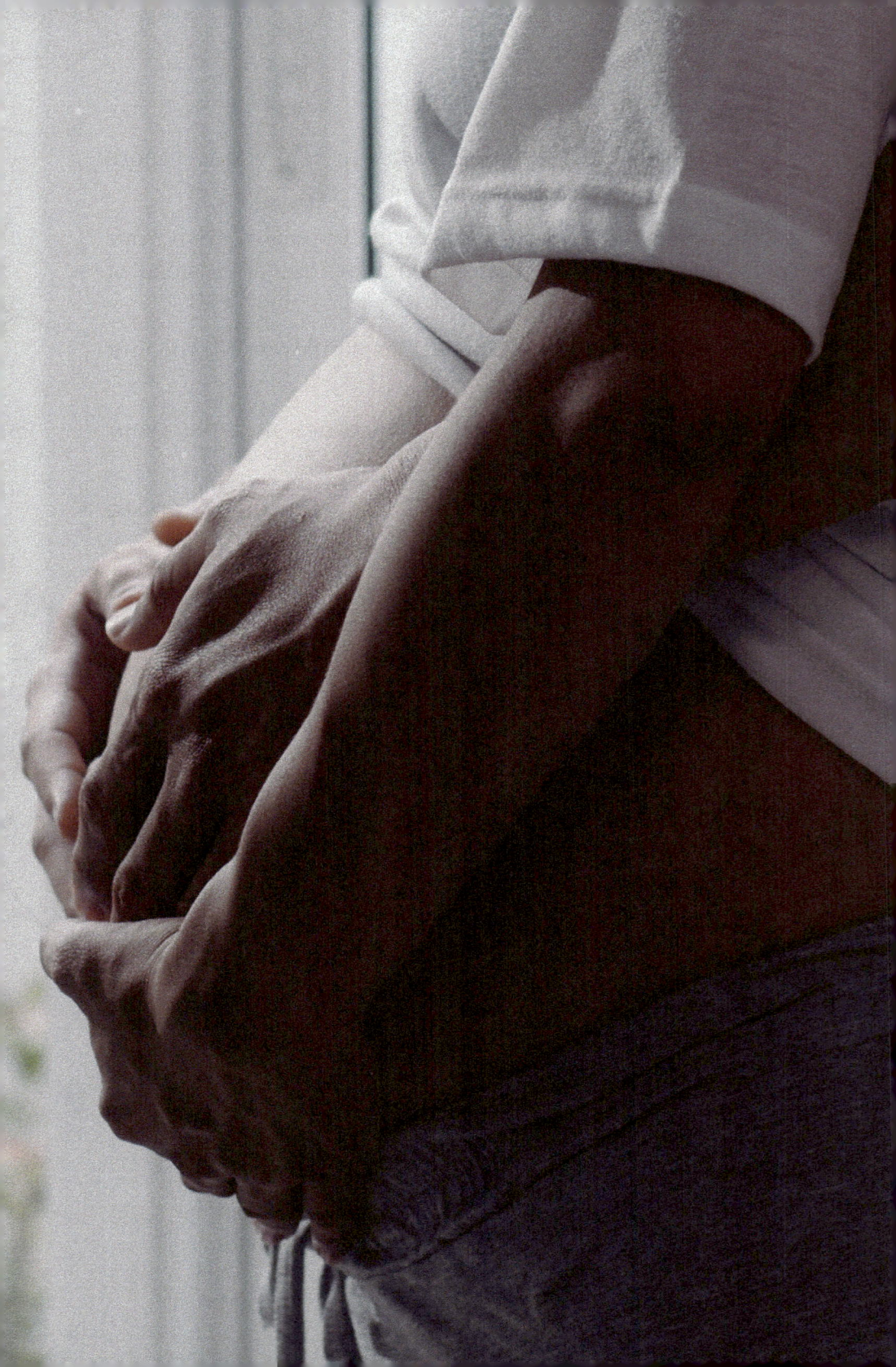

Chapter 7: Getting to Know your Birthing zone

Learning to relax or meditate is a fantastic tool for life and especially important to cultivate in preparation for labor. This mind-body preparation pays off later, as regular practice makes it much easier to go to this relaxed space during labor and is especially helpful for the transition from home to the hospital (if you choose a hospital birth).

It also ensures your body stays relaxed for the entire process, so everything flows smoothly, and you can go into a different state altogether—also referred to as "getting in the zone." It is a vital piece of the puzzle.

Empowered to Rearrange the Furniture!

While creating a relaxed internal environment is the first step to getting in the zone. It is essential to recognize that choosing the right birth conditions where you feel most comfortable. Creating a safe space, no matter where you are in your external environment—is just as crucial for feeling at ease for birth.

It is interesting to note. Mammals will not give birth until they feel completely safe and private, away from any predators. We are no different.

Our external environment impacts our internal state. For instance, the mere sight of the hospital medical equipment made me feel uneasy. To create a safe space, my husband asked the nurses to hide any medical equipment on arrival to the hospital, so I would "feel more at home" (I didn't want to feel like a patient). They thought this was a strange request, but they had no choice but to go along with it.

He then asked them to remove the clock from the wall in the labor ward. It meant I could lose all sense of time and space, instead of clock watching and minimize the distraction of a constant ticking in my ear, while making "getting in the zone" easier.

Thank goodness he did, as I was completely unaware of being in the hospital for the next 12 hours! It would have felt like an eternity, had I known, and would have impacted my confidence.

Thank goodness for the knowledge I had gained from my excellent birth course, as I would never have thought to do any of these things or have the nerve to rearrange the furniture! In essence, I was doing everything in my power to make myself feel comfortable, safe, and create a homely environment in a private hospital.

The Power of Hypnosis and Going to a Happy Place

Testimony by Erika M.:

«How did I get in the zone?

As soon as I set the scene with my husband and the initial monitoring was completed, the first thing I did was lay on the floor on my side with my favorite big soft pillow and cozy blanket from home. I then turned my attention inward, rather than focusing on what was going on around me and listened to my trusty hypnobirthing CD.

It was like an old friend and calmed me instantly. The CD was the same one I had used throughout my pregnancy, so my body responded immediately by going into a deep state of relaxation. It felt like I was going deep within myself into a dream-like state or going to another place. It was all part of the "plan" to ensure everything would proceed normally and not slow down events as I had read about so many times. It worked wonders!

My membranes hadn't broken, but by the time the midwife examined me, I was already almost fully dilated. She said it was too late for any pain relief if I wanted any. My midwife felt there was no point in breaking my membranes as I was already so far along—I wouldn't have wanted them broken artificially anyway.

As I walked into the room, I sat up on the bed. I felt like a zombie, and although my mind was very aware of what was going on, my body was just doing what it was told. I never envisaged I would be on the bed. I thought I would be on my hands and knees in my zone, but I went along with it, and they checked whatever they needed to.

After all of that, my zone had been re-established. While lying on the bed, so I never got up from the ground again. I gave birth on my back in the classic childbirth position you see in the movies!

The midwife kept asking me if I wanted to get up and move around or go onto all fours, and I just knew if I moved, I would get distracted and come out of my zone, so by my own choice, I stayed there!

The midwife called the student midwife who was assisting me and eventually reached my obstetrician once I had begun pushing. At one point, the midwife said to me: "That sounded like you wanted to push." I said I had wanted to since the car. She hadn't realized how far along I was, or it must have progressed quite quickly.

Even though I had confidence in what my body was telling me, I feared tearing and stitches. After a while of pushing by myself, they started talking me through it. The student midwife was the most involved, and when my obstetrician arrived, she stood back and didn't say much.

She let the student have the experience I am grateful for, as she knew me—and what I was hoping for during the birth. She helped me with my breathing during the pushing and telling me to push down into the baby.

During that phase, nurses kept coming in to look, as seeing a baby being born in its membrane was rare.

What helped most during this phase was the midwives, obstetrician, and my mum, who told me after each push they could see his head—and knowing every inspiration was one step closer to him coming out. I think hubby was in a bit of shock during the whole thing and offered encouraging words.

With my sister taking the photos, hubby and mum were able to stay up near me—I held one of their hands the whole time. They kept asking me whether I wanted to have a look in the mirror or feel his head, and surprisingly, I didn't want to because again, as soon as I contemplated doing something different, my zone would get disrupted.

Feeling him, seeing what was going on, and touching him as he came out was something I had wanted to do, but I just couldn't move my body or do anything else other than focus on what I had to do.

Throughout the labor, I was thinking, "This isn't that bad… I'm getting through this." Knowing what part of labor, I was up to and how I was progressing helped get through it. I kept thinking, "These contractions aren't that long."

It must have been a while on the bed, trying not to push through the contractions when my mind started to get a bit tired.

I think I muttered, "I can't," but this was counteracted with the midwife and my mum saying, "You can, and you are doing it."

With every contraction, I was giving a low, long moan. Vocalizing helped me to get through it. There was no screaming, until the push in which the head came out. I didn't realize I had screamed until it happened, and I think I may have laughed afterward.

My mum described it as a "primal animal wail," and it was just an instinctual thing to do. Hubby said he had never heard a scream like that in his life—it was just a sudden, one-off loud yell, which my dad and brother said they could listen to from the waiting area.

As the end was getting nearer, I started to leave my zone and become more aware of my mum, hubby, midwives, and sister. We even have a photo of the midwives. While I was laughing at my sister, she took pictures at the end of the bed, in between pushes.

Bub eventually popped out and was given straight to me. I was told to blow on his face because he was in shock and wasn't taking a breath properly. I wasn't scared because the obstetricians and nurses were calm about it.

They asked who would cut the cord, but I said I wanted to keep the cord connected for a while. They calmly said they needed to cut it because it needed to move him to give him oxygen. I remember them asking if it was okay.

If I said it was important to me for the cord to stay connected, they would have moved the oxygen machine or my bed. Just knowing it was not doing anything without my approval made me feel relieved, and I said, "that's fine,"—and my mum cut the cord.

As they had our baby in the corner on the bed with the oxygen, my husband asked if everything was okay, but I knew everything was fine. They gave the baby back to me, and we watched as he was making his way to my nipple. My mum, a breastfeeding counselor, was there eagerly awaiting the photo of bub latching on by himself!

Eventually, the midwife attached him.

Overall, I'd describe my birthing experience at the hospital as positive. I was lucky enough to have midwives who allowed me to give birth in the way I felt comfortable. I was also fortunate enough to have a quick seven-hour labor and wasn't faced with a situation where any complications challenged the birth I had hoped for.

I think the most important things, which made it possible, were my preparation and mindset in the lead-up, reading and watching positive birthing stories, doing yoga, and keeping active during pregnancy.

I had read about lots of positions and how to cope during labor. In the end, I just did what my body was telling me.

I also believe the raspberry leaf tea I was drinking a few times a day helped with my contractions and strength of my uterus. Also, the support and confidence my midwives and support people showed me during the birth were essential.

I did have a positive birthing experience in the private hospital, but perhaps next time, I'll choose to have my birth in a homier environment of a birth center.»

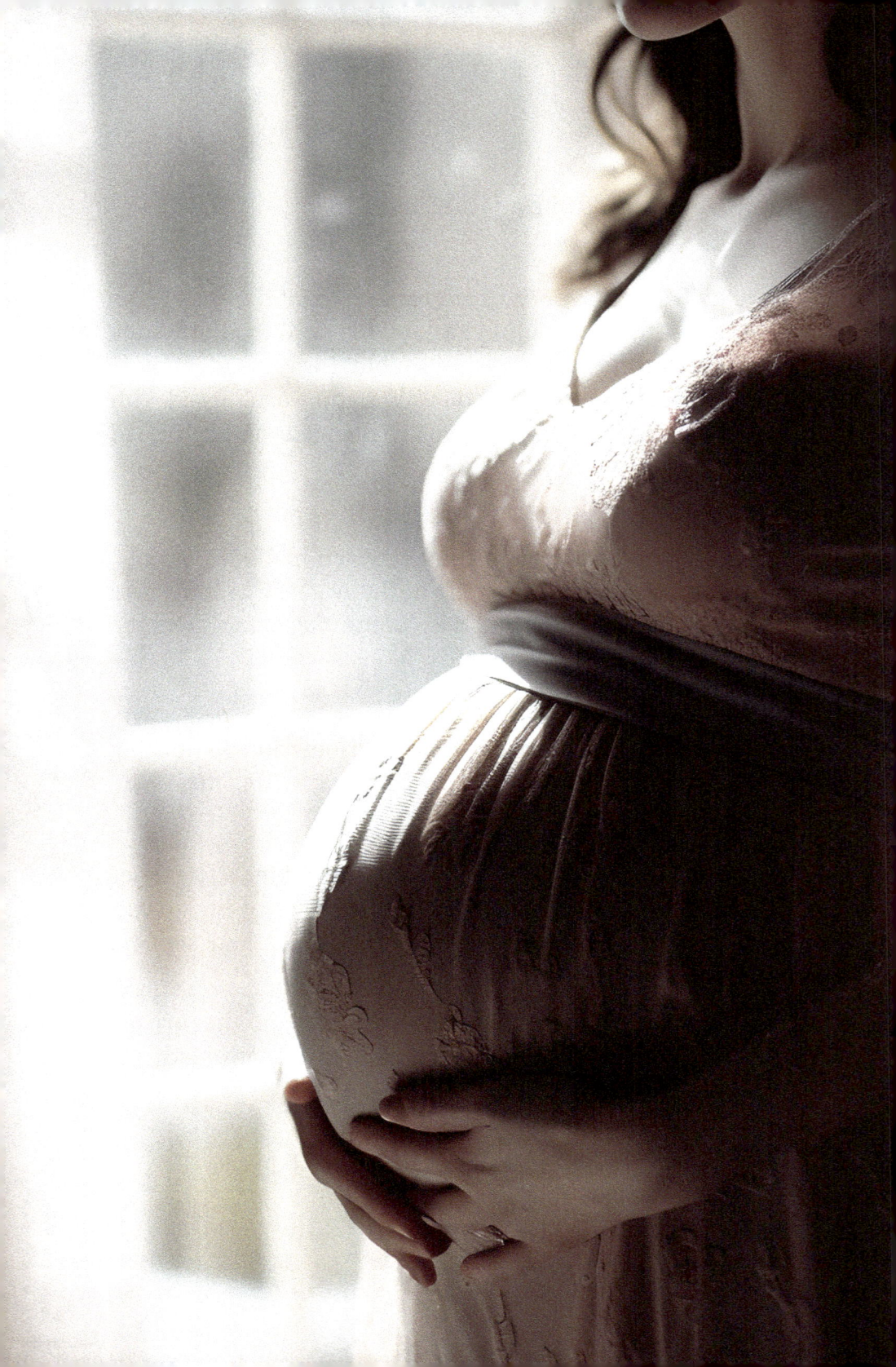

Chapter 8: Letting Go of Fear and Anxiety

Fear of Childbirth

Because you probably already know, there's so much knowledge regarding childbirth from a wide variety of sources that it's no surprise that many people get flustered, puzzled, nervous, depressed, and even terrified of delivery itself.

An article published in the British Journal of Psychiatry in 2000 (2000, 176: 83-85) coined the word 'tokophobia' as the recognized psychological disorder explaining the intense fear of childbirth. Recent studies in Sweden and Finland have culminated in many of their hospitals setting up' fear of childbirth' teams that work on these problems. Their ultimate objective is to make it as satisfying as possible to give birth, whatever the kind of delivery.

While there are no such teams in the UK, there is still something you can do to handle that terror, however small or large it may be. Know, you're not alone, and as labor progresses, many women feel some anxiety, which represents the emotional pregnancy cycle. Sorting through these thoughts while you are breastfeeding helps reduce the stress of having a new baby adjust to life. As the first step in parenthood, it leaves you ready to undergo labor and childbirth.

Who, Instead, Will Help?

Write a journal Writing down your thoughts and emotions will help highlight specific concerns or worries that you have but are not sure what to do about them at this stage. You may choose to enlist the help of someone experienced at birth or in the form of fear that you feel.

Talk to people about your anxiety. It can sometimes make them feel larger than they are when faced with doubts or worries. Do not be embarrassed to ask others if voicing them to your wife, relatives, or a close friend does not improve. An accomplished nurse, doula (a professional qualified to provide emotional and logistical assistance to a woman (or couple) before, during, and after childbirth), birth instructor or psychologist, midwife, or another therapist may help you overcome your birth concerns. Also, it can benefit from having the opportunity to chat openly and honestly.

Antenatal Workshops

Train yourself by learning the basics about childbirth, labor, and delivery, either by reading and educating yourself or by taking a seminar on maternal care. Attending a class allows you to ask questions when they occur, which are relevant to you. Knowledge promotes harmony and preparation, and it will dissipate any doubts you may have made based on misinformation. Seek not to hear the' horror stories' so many people are eager to tell you!

Visit the area you are about to give birth to.

If you are considering a hospital birth but can't go in person, several websites of maternal hospitals also offer online' virtual tours.' Studies have shown that this would help lessen the anxieties and fears. You will give birth in a healthy, efficient, and comfortable atmosphere by getting the right combination of labor hormones.

If you are usually scared of hospitals, Try arranging a birth center or home birth with a qualified midwife. If this is not practical and time is limited for your caregiver, schedule a consultation with a professional midwife, doula, labor advisor, or therapist.

Each of these could help you find a response to your anxiety.

Just as the body knows how to shape a pregnancy, it knows how to give birth. You can have trust in labor by feeling connected to your body. Consider having a monthly massage with a practitioner that has a particular interest in the wellbeing of women. Not only do they cope with aches and pains, but they can also ensure that you are in top condition for a very healthy birth company and allow you to be in contact with your body and infant.

Activity: Regular activity during breastfeeding helps to build the body's sense of confidence. Enrolling in a particular Pilates or yoga class not only helps positively prepare your body and mind, but it can also teach you strategies to deal with the birth conditions that can be imposed on your body. Swimming or aqua natal lessons are also suitable to exercise types, as you do not put any pressure on your joints.

Deep relaxation techniques: Consider attending a specific course designed to teach you about the strategies of self-hypnosis, hypnobirthing, guided meditation, imagination, or mindfulness, or deep relaxation. There are now several courses available which were developed by experts, specially designed for birth.

Caregiver help and consistency: You may be less scared because you know you won't be alone at practice. Recent studies show that patients accompanied by doulas or midwives benefit from faster labors, lower epidural anesthesia levels, and fewer births in the cesarean section. Consider, if possible, the choice of having a doula or enlisting an experienced midwife's help to ensure continuity of care and encouragement during delivery. If this is not necessary, pick careers and nurses who will be with you throughout the birth process. Make sure that everybody invited to your birth accepts the choices that you have made. Surround yourself with people who are now motivated and emotional support.

Birth arrangements & the ability to take charge: Just as birth isn't just something that's happening to you, giving birth isn't something you're doing. Create and share your dream birth plan with your parents, and they learn your project and the reasoning behind your desires. Getting trained like this gives you confidence even before the birth process begins, so you've made the best possible decisions for you. You will start building a good working relationship by addressing it with your parents, which will proceed throughout the birthing process. When unforeseen situations arise, make sure that you are part of the decision-making process, decide how to continue.

These are some of the items that you can do now to help you resolve labor worries. Choose the resources that you think will work well for you and focus for a week or two on them. Remember the anxiety again when you have achieved this; do you need to make more changes or do more research to resolve your fears? Take the time to investigate any doubt you may have. The first step towards a natural birth is to overcome the fear of labor.

Overcoming Fear in Pregnancy and Childbirth

Pregnancy can be a period of fear, particularly if you don't know the options that are available to you. Confronting your fears, coping with them, and making wise choices, is critical. Anxiety itself can have an emotionally and physically crippling effect that, if not well controlled, can be detrimental to you, your baby, and your whole birth experience.

If "the reality will set you free" is valid, instead, information can be the answer to terror. Fear, coupled with a lack of knowledge, could in three ways impede our best efforts. It may paralyze us in embracing our conclusions, which may or may not be factually based. It can drive us into bad choices, unconsciously clouding our brains so that rationality cannot prevail. And finally, irrational anxiety of pregnancy and childbirth can have physical effects that lead to complications, avoid recovery, and render birth more painful than it should be.

It is, therefore, crucial for you and your baby's well-being that you take the time to face your fears and cope with them early on in your path. One way to do that is to look at all the choices. For starters, if you fear the actual process of childbirth, start by learning what happens during that period. The internet or parenting workshop will show you what your body is doing to get your baby into this universe. It is quite impressive.

Know what to expect from each of the three stages of work and the different strategies to manage each.

Find out about your choices, in addition to the physical labor information. Were you planning on birth at a hospital because that's what everyone you know did? What are the advantages of a local birth center or home birth? See how the theory, method, and skills of midwives vary from ob.-gyms. There's a lot to learn but getting the information that can ease your worries and help you make informed choices for yourself and your baby is worth it.

Another critical step in coping with anxiety could include a session to relieve fear. This technique should assist in overcoming perceptions that need more than mere facts.

Hypnobirthing is one form of childbirth therapy that helps your pregnancy take an internal inventory and confront the worries that might impede you. If not treated, a few hurts and insecurities from your history may interfere with the birth process. The concerns must be remembered and set free somehow, such as putting them on paper and burning them away. It can boost your mental and emotional health, and the body can do its job. Of course, some more personal severe anxieties and issues can require professional counseling.

Knowledge may not fix all of your pregnancy's challenges, dilemmas, and hang-ups, but it can bring you comfort and trust in making wise choices at every level, allowing you to do the best you can for yourself and your kid. Try to be objective and know everything you can, then set aside your prejudices. It probably shocked you. Best still, you may be released.

How to Keep Staying Positive?

Natural birth is what all pregnant women aim for, maybe they don't know, but they do. We're just scared to say we're GOING to have a natural birth for fear of the product not falling in! I hear to convey to you this way of thinking is just how you get the delivery you don't want!

You've heard of the saying: "What you're focused on is growing," I appreciate this and deal with it every day. What we don't know is that it will multiply, whether we concentrate on the good or the bad. It can be extended to the way we feel when pregnant and on our path to childbirth. So, is it so straightforward to just stay positive?

No, that isn't it!!

Have you ever passed through the grocery store, your big belly pressing against the trolley, and a woman came up to you, smiling and saying, "When are you due?" You grin and answer her; this somehow turns into, "Please tell me your horror story, when I'm exhausted, upset, and already terrified!!!" We've all been there, and we hate it, so why do we hear it repeatedly.

That sort of negative conversation is what regular pregnant women must deal with, not just their feelings, but that of the public! We will bite our tongue as non-pregnant women, or tell a lovely birth story, or even just say, "You look beautiful" and leave it at that.

If we don't fill our minds with positive self-talk, then someone will do it for us!! So, ladies, fill your head with all the pretty things you want from your natural birth, particularly how you want it to end.

Chapter 9: Techniques

Relaxation Techniques

In Yoga, we learn how the mind and bodywork together. We know how to relax the body and silence the mind. A crucial part of this learning process is understanding the importance of our breathing. Breathing through the mouth is such a waste of energy - yet this is how so many people live daily. It is sometimes recognized as panic breathing.

Busy lifestyles can cause us to rush around and pay little attention to our breath. Watch a sleeping baby and notice how his/her chest rises with each inhale and deflates with each exhale. You will also see that he/she is most likely breathing through the nose. It is done instinctively. Nobody teaches a baby how to breathe.

It is doubtful that a baby is rushing around the place of panic breathing, as most adults do. It was never nature's intention for us to breathe through our mouth. But when we get into the habit of panic breathing through our mouth, we sometimes forget to go back to breathing correctly - through our nose.

While doing any form of exercise, it is recommended to breathe through the nose. It is to save energy and to improve the effectiveness of the training. It's the same concept in labor. It's never too late in the pregnancy to learn how to breathe correctly, but the earlier you start practicing, the better. Taking time to sit and focus on your breathing is also a fantastic form of meditation.

It is called conscious breathing. While you are entirely focused on inhaling and exhaling, your mind is taking a break from thinking about all the everyday issues or problems that cause most of us to feel stressed.

Learning how to breathe effectively will become part of your plan for a healthy pregnancy and pain-free natural birth. Allow yourself fifteen minutes every day to practice conscious breathing.

Find a nice, quiet place where you won't be disturbed (No phone zone). Sit in a comfortable position making sure your back is straight. Close your eyes and, keeping your mouth closed, bring your full attention to your breath. Don't force anything but simply feel the air coming in through your nose and as you exhale, feel the air leaving your nose. Become aware that you are breathing naturally and with ease.

Feel how your tummy and chest inflates with each inhale and then feel them deflating as you exhale. Just like a balloon expanding as it is filled with air and then shrinks as the air leaves it. Notice the warm air leaving your nostrils as you exhale.

It's essential to allow all thoughts to come to you and know that your busy mind during this meditation only indicates that stress is leaving you now. As your ideas come to you, acknowledge them, and then allow them to pass. Continue to focus on your breath, and you will eventually feel a peace come over you.

It is the moment when your mind has given up thinking and becomes relaxed following your body. Your mind and body are at one at this moment, and it is here that you can experience the healing of both. After about ten or fifteen minutes, open your eyes, and notice how relaxed you have become. You may also feel refreshed and uplifted.

If you practice conscious breathing like this regularly, you will become more relaxed and calmer throughout your day for more extended periods. You will notice that you are more centered and self-confident, even in the most stressful times. It is a potent exercise that aims to restore your body and mind, essentially bringing you back to zero. Meditation exercises are best done in the morning and evening time on an empty stomach.

Visualization Techniques

Creative Visualization is essentially a technique to help you create what you want, whether that's more love, peace, fulfillment, self-expression, money, or anything else you want in your life! It is the process of using your thought ability to deliberately envision, create, and entice to yourself the things that you intend to experience in your life. Mastering creative visualization gives you direct control over your thoughts at a subconscious level.

You can become happier, more relaxed, more focused, mentally stronger, and more peaceful through your practice of Creative Visualization. You'll get more of what you want, but you'll also feel more positive about life in general.

Visualization includes discovering and altering your earnest outlooks to life. It can have a reflective effect on you and those around you! Visualization is well "mental rehearsal." It means that you exercise roughly in your mind, rather than physically.

By imagining tasks, you want to do in the future, and you can increase your skill-level, all with the power of your mind! Several scientific studies show that mental rehearsal improves physical skill, comprising firing basketball free-throws, enhancing your golf swing, and growing exam scores, and, of course, having a natural, comfortable, pain-free birth.

Though there are numerous ways to program the subconscious mind, visualization is one of the most effective and produces quick outcomes.

Scientists are beginning to share the same belief as spiritual and metaphysical teachers. They believe that our physical universe is primarily composed of energy. They teach us that physically, we are all made up of power, and we are all a part of the same giant field of energy. Everything is made up of different forms of life that vibrate at a different speed.

It is believed that all forms of energy are interconnected in some way. Similar types will attract each other. Our thoughts and feelings will attract the life that is of a similar structure. When we think happy thoughts, we attract feelings of happiness. Our physical appearance becomes a happy one.

When we think angry thoughts, we become mad and then show physical signs of anger. Our thoughts manifest into actions. By thinking of a specific nature when visualizing, you are more likely to "attract" this experience energetically. The more you practice creative visualization, the faster you will create the life you want.

The visualization techniques drawn here will aid you in attaching the creative power of your thoughts to modify your situations and deliberately create the life you desire. Of course, visualization is by no means a magic wand. If you visualize being offered the job of your dreams, you must be trained in the skills required to do the job in question, and you must be actively job searching.

Nobody gets offered their dream job by sitting at home watching television 24/7. Your visualization practices will attract opportunities on which you must act. The same goes for visualizing a pain-free natural birth. You must be prepared to put in a little bit of effort to prepare yourself physically and mentally for the day your baby makes his or her entrance into the world.

How to Use Visualization in Your Life

Your brain produces five different types of brainwaves, Gamma, beta, alpha, theta, and delta. Each class is related to varying states of consciousness. During times of high mental activity such as studying or problem-solving, your brain is producing gamma waves. Less intense mental activities such as concentrating on tasks and active processing have beta waves.

Alpha waves are produced when you are in a relaxed and happy state but very much awake and alert. When you are comfortable, and in an intense meditative state or REM sleep, theta waves are produced. The slowest of all five is the Delta waves, and they occur when you are in a night of quiet dreamless sleep.

Visualization is much more effective when your brainwaves are in alpha because you have much better access to your subconscious mind and emotions. It is when you can easily create vivid and compelling Visualizations.

By practicing the breathing exercises outlined, You Have the Power to Relax.

You should ideally be able to put yourself into a state of relaxation that will cause your brain to produce alpha waves if this is a challenging exercise for you.

Chapter 10: Breathing Technique

Diminishing sensations during labor can make your introduction to the world simpler, faster, and more settled, yet is this conceivable? It is! You can decrease feelings during your works with the correct breathing systems.

Luckily, with enough practice and tutelage, you can. Why? It is because you'd have to inhale profoundly to loosen up your muscles and leave your uterus free of strain. It will assist you in taking care of and oversee agony and worry during your introduction to the world.

Flood Breathing

The point when you experience your floods or withdrawals, you don't need to remember muddled strategies. You just need to recall breathing examples that are now normal to your body.

Flood breathing is stomach relaxing. All through each flood, you must inhale equally and profoundly, breathing down into your midriff, feeling it rise and grow.

In unwinding breathing, you figure out how to quiet yourself, and it doesn't make a difference where you inhale into. In flood breathing, it's critical to inhale into your stomach or guts. There are a few people who regularly inhale into their bellies. Other people inhale into their chests. Thus, it's critical to watch your breathing examples.

Do this speedy exercise: Place one hand on your chest and another on your stomach. Unwind as much as you can and put power or exertion into your relaxing. Simply see where your breathing goes.

On the off chance that you routinely profound into your chest, your rib confines agreements, and it requires you more vitality and exertion to move those ribs upward. Along these lines, during a flood, when you inhale into your gut, your breath gets increasingly slow. You use less vitality and get more oxygen. The more oxygen you inhale into your tummy through the flood, the better for you, your muscles, and your infant.

Decrease in Stress

When you do flood breathing, you extend your mid-region and lungs, which gives the vertical muscles of your uterus more space to reach down and pull up the roundabout muscles. This additional space for your uterus muscles decreases the power of the flood and makes it simpler to oversee.

The more you inhale into your belly, the simpler the weight impressions of the flood will be for you. Try not to be scared by stomach breathing in case you're accustomed to living into your chest. Have you seen resting babies of late? They inhale with their stomachs. Stomach breathing will come to you usually. You simply need some training.

Calm Breathing

It is anything but an unprecedented sight for and anticipating that mum should frenzy and feel terrified of work, mainly a first-time mum. The latter has heard every one of the anecdotes about agonizing births. Usually, when she begins shouting, the specialist or medical caretaker says, "Relax. Simply relax. You have to quiet down."

At the point when you're pushed or apprehensive, it's never simple to quiet down, to unwind, and to inhale appropriately. It's troublesome, yet not feasible. With hypnobirthing, you can relax and inhale tranquility to remove the weight from your body, to lighten the torment during work.

With the Hypnobirthing Hub, you can utilize unwinding breathing methods, which will assist you with resisting the urge to panic and loose during your pregnancy, through your floods, and during your work. This breathing procedure is perfect for the beginning or pre-work stages and in the middle of floods to enable you to unwind. The more you relax, the more your muscles will disengage, the simpler your work will be.

Unwinding breathing is something beyond working on breathing in and breathing out. All in all, how is it done?

Do this short exercise:

Close your eyes, take a long breath in, and afterward, a long breath out. Do you discover the in-breath or out-breath more unwinding?

Since out-breathing or breathing out is more unwinding, you will concentrate on this more when you do unwind relaxing. Your out-breath will be twice the length of your in-breath.

Unwinding Between Your Surges

In the middle of your compressions is when dread and uneasiness sneaks in. Indeed, even a spur of the moment remark questioning your capacity to deal with the floods or a doubting glance toward you can make you begin to feel terrified and on edge.

Since we birth like well-evolved creatures and have such a necessary reaction at our birthing time, our impulses are excessively elevated, and we feel incredibly delicate.

You can't control everybody and everything around you during your introduction to the world, yet you can manage your very own feelings and make a feeling of quiet at whatever point you need it. If you ever feel you could do some additional unwinding between your floods, simply take a couple of unwinding breaths, and feel restored and sure again.

Unwinding Breathing Technique

Enable your eyelids to delicately close.

Deliberately drop and loosen up your jaw, neck, and entire

body.

Gradually breathe in through your nose (or mouth) to the check of four. Take in 1,2,3,4.

Rehash multiple times or as expected to feel superbly loose.

Surge Breathing

Designed breathing alludes to the demonstration of breathing at any number of possible rates and profundities. A few ladies incline toward living profoundly, utilizing their stomach to fill their guts with air. Other ladies lean toward light breathing, breathing in only enough to fill their chest. The objective is to discover breathing designs that have a quieting and loosening up impact. Your breathing ought to be at an agreeable rate and ought not to make you feel shy of breath or unsteady.

The more you find out about work and birth, the more you will perceive how various examples of breathing are utilized at different stages. You will find out about using breathing to concentrate on making every compression a valuable piece of the birthing procedure. Whether pregnant or not, designed breathing is useful in adapting to different kinds of agony, inconvenience, tension, and dread.

Advantages of rehearsing designed relaxing:

- Breathing turns into a programmed reaction to torment
- The mother stays in an increasingly loosened upstate

and will react more decidedly to the beginning of torment

- The enduring musicality of breathing is quieting during work

- Gives a feeling of prosperity and control

- Expanded oxygen provides more quality and vitality to both the mother and child

- Carries reason to every withdrawal, making constrictions progressively gainful

- Congested driving conditions, cerebral pains, and family unit tasks give chances to rehearse distinctive breathing methods and make them part of your everyday practice. To recreate work, some labor instructors recommend grasping an ice block while rehearsing effective breathing methods.

- Toward the start and end of every compression, make sure to take a profound, purifying, loosening up breath. It hones your concentration and gives more oxygen to your infant, your muscles, and your uterus.

- Breathing designs for the principal phase of work.

Slow Breathing

Start moderate breathing when withdrawals are severe enough that you can never again walk or talk through them without stopping. Utilize moderate relaxing for whatever length of time that you think that it's accommodating. Change to another example on the off chance that you become tense and never again unwind during compressions.

Take a sorting out a breath, a prominent murmur when the withdrawal starts. Release all pressure (limp all finished – from head to toe) as you inhale out.

Concentrate.

Gradually breathe in through your nose. Then breathe out through your mouth, enabling all your air to stream out with a murmur. Respite until the atmosphere appears to "need" to come in once more.

With each breathes out, center around loosening up an alternate piece of your body (see Relaxation Techniques).

Light Accelerated Breathing

Most ladies want to change to light breathing eventually during the busy period of work. Give the force of your withdrawals a chance to control you in choosing when to utilize soft relaxing. Take in and out quickly out of your mouth at about one breath for each second. Maintain your breathing thin and light. Your inward breaths ought to be peaceful, yet your exhalation perceptible.

Take a sorting out-breath—a prominent murmur when the compression begins. Discharge all pressure (limp all completed – from head to toe) as you inhale out.

Breathe in gradually through your nose and breathe out through your mouth. Quicken and help your breathing as the compression increments in force. On the off chance that the compression tops early, at that point, you should quicken from the get-go in the constriction. It if tops more step by step, you will work up to top speed more gradually.

Keep your mouth and shoulders loose.

As the withdrawal diminishes in force, continuously moderate your breathing rate, exchanging back to taking in through your nose and out through your mouth.

At the point when the compression closes, take your completing breath—breathe out with a murmur.

Variable (Transition) Breathing

It is a variety of light relaxing. Another it is, in some cases, alluded to as "gasp blow" or "hee-hee-who" comfortable. Variable breathing joins week, shallow breathing with an occasional longer or increasingly articulated exhalation. Irregular breathing is utilized in the principal organize if you feel overpowered, incapable to unwind, despondently, or depleted.

Take a sorting out-breath—a prominent murmur when the constriction starts. Release all pressure (limp all completed – from head to toe) as you inhale out.

When the withdrawal closes, take a couple of deep loosening up breaths with a moan.

Breathing to abstain from pushing at an inappropriate time

There will be times all through the two phases of work when you need to push or weigh down. However, it isn't the ideal time. Most ladies need to hold their breath during these, especially troublesome minutes. Abstain from holding your breath by taking in and out continually or by raising your jaw and blowing or gasping. It shields you from adding to the pushing that your body is as of now doing.

Breathing designs for the second phase of work.

Removal Breathing

They are utilized once the cervix is wholly enlarged, and the second phase of work has started.

Take a sorting out-breath—a major moan when the compression starts. Terminate all pressure (limp all finished – from head to toe) as you inhale out.

Concentrate on the infant going disheartened, or on another positive picture.

Inhale gradually, giving the constriction a chance to control you. Quicken or help your breathing as vital for comfort. At the point when you can't fight the temptation to push (when it is "requests" that you participate), take a significant breath, fold your jaw to chest, twist your body and fit forward. At that point hunker down, while holding your breath or gradually discharging air by snorting or groaning.

Generally significant of all, loosen up the pelvic floor. Help the child descend by discharging any pressure in the perineum.

At the point when the compression closes, loosen up your body and take a couple of quiet breaths.

Creating Positive Birth Beliefs

You have decided in your heart that you want to give birth the natural way to have the spiritual experience of producing another life and bonding with it. This little human being is frail and fragile, and your maternal instincts will kick in so that you will do everything to protect it. Without this instinct, humans would have been extinct a long time ago. Having a natural birth will give you a greater appreciation for the perpetuation of human life.

There are certain things that you will need to do to prepare yourself for the task of natural childbirth. You will not receive any drugs during labor, and you probably should minimize the medicines you take during pregnancy. Take supplements if you must, but only the essentials such as Vitamin K. Natural childbirth starts from inception, so make sure you have a healthy diet. Pregnancy classes aren't essential, but they will help you learn things you will need to do during pregnancy and childbirth. These classes usually teach labor pain management techniques, which you can use to prepare yourself. These classes are typically held at hospitals and health clinics, but other places have these classes for women and their partners.

You must keep in shape and control your weight gain. Studies have shown that women who are not overweight have fewer complications, requiring less medical intervention. The pregnancy classes mentioned above may also provide exercise classes for pregnant women as well. Swimming and water exercises, specifically for pregnant women, are relaxing and toning at the same time. Ensure that whatever you do, it is conducive to your condition. You should not go sprinting when you're eight months pregnant, for example. Exercise should be done in moderation. Exercise is essential for proper blood flow, and you will need better blood flow to your uterus to experience less pain.

Don't take showers, take baths. Make sure you put yourself in the most comfortable position, the position you would be in when giving birth. Make the water warm, but not too warm, and stay there and relax for about 20 minutes each day. The warm water helps the muscles in the uterus and vagina to function better so that you don't experience too much pain during pregnancy and childbirth. This hydrotherapy method is the reason why a lot of mothers opt for the water-birthing route.

Breathe. Ensure that you take regular and calculated breaths. Put yourself into a relaxed state every day. The best time to do this is during your bath times. Your classes will also teach you how to breathe to help reduce the pain that you may experience.

Find a childbirth educator who will tell you all about natural childbirth and what you should and should not do. Just because you're going natural does not mean you should restrict visits to your doctor. You should go for regular checkups and remind your doctor that you want to take as few drugs as possible. However, if you must take medication for any complication, please do so. Having a natural birth isn't worth it if it means putting your baby at risk. It is also good to talk to a counselor or psychologist who will help you eliminate all the fears you may have. Your worries will hinder your mental preparation for the task ahead, so it is essential to minimize them or get rid of them completely.

You will only compound your fears if you listen to negative stories about natural childbirth. Yes, there are negative aspects to it, and you will need to know them, but listening to negative stories will only put doubts in your mind and worsen your fears. Make sure that you talk to your partner about all your concerns. It is important to tell your partner that he/she is needed to provide a favorable environment for you to bring your child into. Your partner should be your cheerleader.

The pain that accompanies childbirth is more than some women can handle, so they opt for anesthesia. But if you are reading this, it means that you have it in you to go the natural route, even if you may have some reservations about it all. One of the best ways to manage your pain is through mental preparation. This preparation involves getting rid of all the fears that you may be having and using techniques such as hypnosis. It doesn't have to be a scary experience, and you will be relieved to know that there are many ways to reduce the pain that will come with labor.

One way you can reduce the pain is to consider the other methods of giving natural birth rather than going entirely innate, such as a water birth or hypnobirthing. With water births, you are putting yourself into a very relaxed state. The temperature of the water not only eases the muscles in your vagina and uterus, but it also relaxes your mind as well. You don't have to give birth in the water, though. When you are experiencing your first labor pains, you could take a water bath until you are ready to go to the hospital. There are hospitals in the US that offer water births if you are not comfortable having one at home. With hypnobirthing, you are putting your mind into a relaxed state without the aid of outside tools and mediums. With the help of breathing, hypnobirthing takes the mind away from the pain and makes your mind even more receptive to the 'miracle' taking place.

Another way of preparing your mind for childbirth is acceptance. When you accept things the way they are, then you can prepare for the events to come. If you acknowledge that you have a child and that the process of giving life is not easy, then you set your mind at ease. It will help create a relaxed state, which reduces the pain. Acceptance is a spiritual experience that is heightened when you see your baby for the first time. If you are religious, read the scriptures and texts about the beauty of human life, and remind yourself of those scriptures.

Finally, breathe. It was stated that breathing is essential in regularizing blood flow. Breathing takes your body and minds out of the fight and flight state, causing blood to flow away from the uterus, inducing more pain. To prevent that, you must breathe adequately and learn breathing techniques.

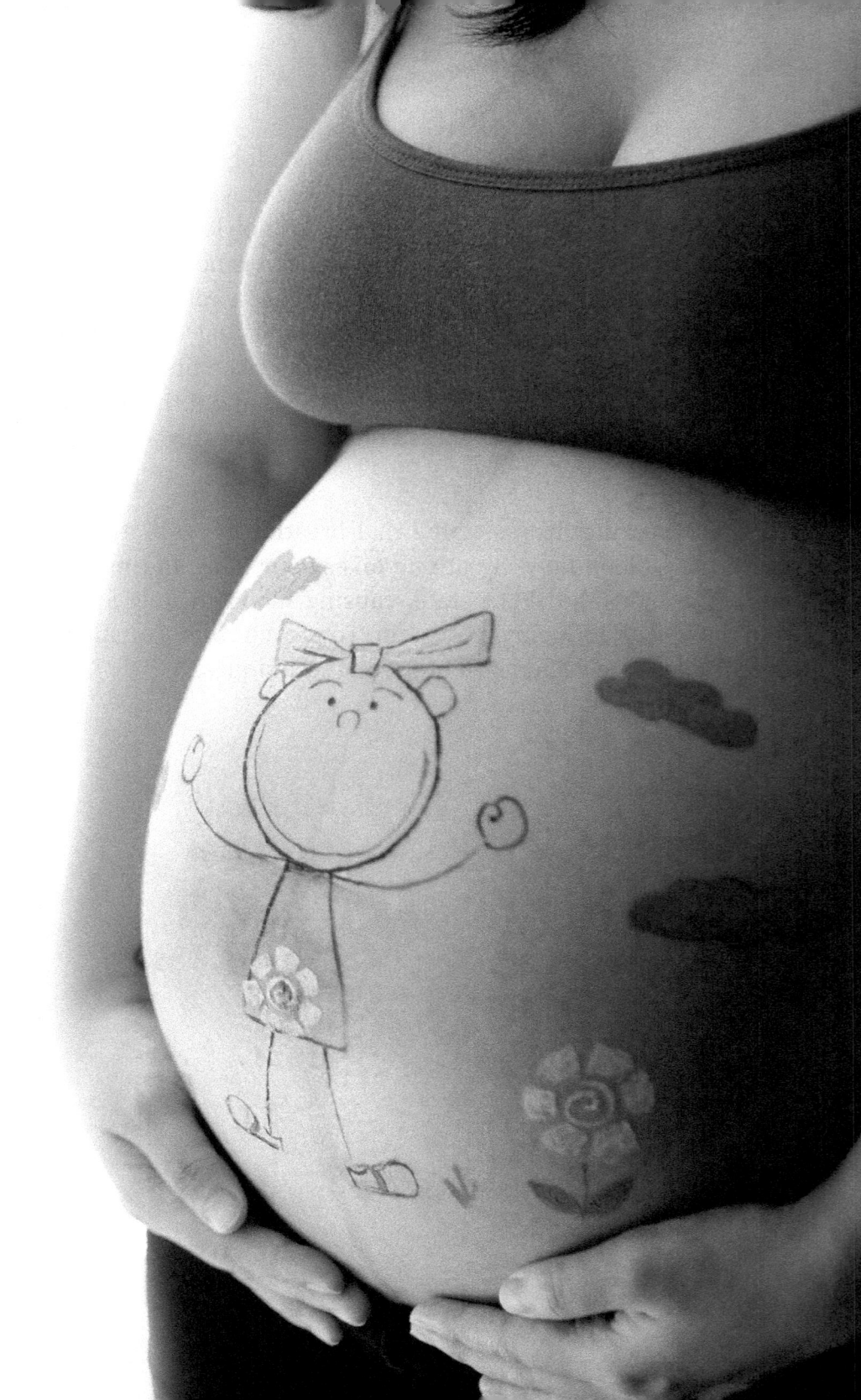

Chapter 11: The Power of Visualization for Birth

If you have neither, ask someone to read this part to you, at least until you know the routine by heart. If you must read and visualize, you might not get the best out of practice.

Choose a relaxing time for your visualization routine. If you already practice antenatal yoga or Tai Chi, you might decide to do this after your exercise routine. It is, however, beneficial to do the visualization routine just before going to bed. It allows the subconscious mind to keep working on these images, making assimilation a lot faster.

Get yourself into a comfortable sitting position. You can play your selected music that relaxes you. It will help your mind to associate the music with relaxation when you are in labor. You might also decide to use the candle or fragrance which you intend to use during your labor.

Close your eyes. You want to see only with the eyes of your mind. Relax your body by taking deep breaths in and out, feel the air you breathe in, reaching each part of your body down to your toes and fingers. Let your stomach expand and deflate with each breath; feel your lungs inflate and deflate with each breath. After a few times, this should get you relaxed but not sleepy! You are now going to use all the tools and information that you have already collected.

1st stage of Labor

Imagine your mucus plug has been expelled, and you are beginning to feel mild contractions. You are in the early stages of labor. The muscles of your cervix are beginning to thin and dilate. Imagine it opening slowly, but surely, millimeters at a time. It is painful.

Imagine that you have gone to boil some water to put in your hot water bottle, or you have started heating your heat pack. You are now lying down and placing the bottle or container on your lower abdomen or back, and you can feel the heat is soothing your pains. After a while, you try to have a warm bath.

Imagine as the pain is now getting a little more robust, and you are pacing the floor of your home. Deeply breathe as you visualize this and say, "I am going to meet my baby soon." "My cervix is opening to let my baby out." "My cervix is working hard." See yourself timing your contractions.

Your contractions are getting stronger. It has reached the stage where you have been advised to send for your midwife. Another option is to go to the hospital. See yourself perform that action. If you plan to have your baby in the hospital or birthing unit, see yourself get into the car and go to the hospital. If you have been told you might have to wait before going into the delivery suite, catch yourself and birthing partner in the waiting room. You are breathing slowly to relax, and you are timing your contractions.

See yourself being ushered into the delivery suite. Take a deep breath and imagine your birthing room. Remember, you already have a good idea of what it will look like. Take a few moments to take in the furniture, the bed, and the walls. See your birthing partner setting up the room with your items, such as the music, the flowers, the fragrances, or even pictures.

Take a few moments to imagine the music playing, take a deep breath to smell the fragrances, and allow your senses to take in your surroundings. Imagine yourself sitting on a birth ball, if you choose to use one, or sitting on the bed. You could also be kneeling on the floor or the bed.

By this time, your contractions are getting much more substantial, your cervix is dilating, and you are now in established labor.

Imagine yourself breathing through your contractions and saying, "my body is working very hard," "my body knows what it is doing," "my cervix is working hard millimeter by millimeter to bring my baby to me."

Imagine the support of your birthing partner, who is either holding you, rubbing your back, or anything you want them to do.

2nd Stage

See your cervix fully dilated to 10cm, and your baby is now ready to come out. Imagine you are feeling contractions and the urge to push. Visualize yourself, bringing your baby out. Tell yourself, "I can now actively bring my baby out." "I can help my body in the process of birthing my baby." "These contractions are bringing my baby closer."

The midwife or doctor asks you to push, and with each push, you can feel your baby descend slowly and smoothly through the birth canal. Imagine taking deep breaths between each push.

Imagine feeling your baby's head pressing on your vagina, and with another push, the head is crowning! A couple more pushes, and your baby's head is finally out!

Soon your baby is entirely out and is placed on your chest. Visualize holding your baby and welcoming him or her to your family. Tell your baby how you have been waiting to meet him/her.

3rd Stage

As you hold your baby, your body is getting back into shape, and your uterus is contracting to expel the placenta. Congratulate your body on a job well done while the contractions are taking place. Your body has worked hard over the last nine months to grow your baby, and now it is returning successfully to how it used to be. It is now beginning its healing process. You might be asked to push or cough so that the placenta can be expelled fully and successfully.

Visualize yourself being taken care of by the midwife and doctors. They clean you and your baby. You might be transferred to a different room after delivery (you can find out if this is usually the case when you do your test run). Imagine your baby boy or girl lying next to you in a little cot, and you are resting in your bed.

You are now a proud mum!

To complete the visualization process, take a deep breath and say to yourself, "I am a proud mum, my body and my baby know exactly what to do." "I am holding my beautiful baby in my arms." "We are both healthy and happy!"

Turn off the music, extinguish the fragrance, and go to sleep with these happy and positive thoughts!

Visualizing what is taking place during labor is also vital to help you cope with labor pains. Start from when your cervix begins to dilate. It moves through to established labor and the bearing downstage, and finish with the expelling of the placenta. Since you know what is happening in your body, you can picture it.

However, if you wait until labor to start visualizing the birth process, the pain you will be experiencing will make the technique more difficult to carry out. Visualize this process many times before actual delivery so that your mind gets to know the picture you are presenting to it with, as this will help block the pain signals that your body is sending.

Involving your birth partner

It is always a good idea to involve the person(s) who will be with you during the delivery. When labor starts, it might be more challenging to remember all the things you have mastered. If you have spent enough time learning the visualization techniques, you will find that it might come to you more naturally. However, during labor itself, it will be useful to have someone remind you of certain things, such as your breathing, affirmations, etc.

To make fair use of your birth partner in this process, it is best to decide beforehand what you want them to do and when. For instance, you could ask them to remind you to both breathe properly and think of the beautiful baby you will be having, or anything else you have discovered that might be useful for your visualization. It could be as simple as helping you to set up the room exactly the way you want it to be. Be as specific as possible in explaining what you want. It will ensure that you can get the exact help that you need.

Of course, there are other things your birth partner(s) can do for you apart from aiding your visualization techniques. These could include massage to relieve some of the labor pain, talking to the midwife or doctor on your behalf, helping you move around, etc.

Chapter 12: What is a Birth Plan, and Why is it Important?

Whether you're giving birth in the hospital, at home, or a birth center, creating a birth plan is an essential part of having the birth experience you want. It is an excellent opportunity to research all your options and discuss them with your partner and your care provider.

It can also help you and your birth partner to communicate your desires when the intensity and excitement of labor and birth make it impossible for you to do so yourself.

Hospital Birth Plan

Your birth plan can act as speaking points for reviewing your planned hospital birth with your care provider at your prenatal arrangements. You also need to be able to convey your birth plan with altering shifts of nurses, on-call doctors, and hospital teams that you may have never met before, and that may or may not contribute to your birth philosophy. It would be impractical to convey your birth plan to each of them orally while coping with contractions. Instead, offering them copies of your birth plan can help communicate for you.

Hospital birth plans tend to be more focused on avoiding

interventions because they are readily available and commonly used in that setting.

Sample Hospital Birth Plan

Here's an example of a hospital birth plan from Anjanette's planned hospital birth. Just keep in mind that every birth plan is highly individual.

If possible, I wish to have a:

- Vaginal Delivery
- Without pain medication or anesthesia of any kind
- In the presence of family and my doula

Labor and Delivery:

During labor, I would like:
- My husband to be present the entire time
- To eat and drink if I feel like it
- To shower or bathe for relaxation
- To labor in whatever position feels comfortable
- As few vaginal exams as possible
- To be able to move around without an IV attached (heparin lock is fine)
- Intermittent fetal monitoring preferred

- To wear my clothing

I would like to avoid:

- An Episiotomy
- An IV unless emergency
- Induction via Pitocin, membrane stripping/rupture, or any other method without my consent.
- Cesarean section
- Epidural (or any other anesthesia without consent)

In case of an emergency, I would like:

- To have all procedures explained to my husband and me ahead of time
- To get a second opinion before induction or cesarean
- To remain conscious and with my husband
- To stay with the baby always

Postpartum and Recovery:

Immediately after delivery, I would like:

- The cord to be clamped and only cut after it stops pulsing
- To hold the baby right away (before weighing or washing)
- To breastfeed right away (before considering or passing)
- To deliver the placenta spontaneously and without manual assistance or Pitocin if possible

We would like to decline:

- Vitamin K
- Antibiotic eye ointment
- Vaccinations
- Any other tests or procedures without our consent

Please do not give the baby:

- Bottles
- Formula or sugar water
- Pacifiers

We would like to:

- Room in with our baby
- Breastfeed on demand
- Be discharged as early as possible if we feel well

Out-of-Hospital Birth Plan

If you're preparing an out-of-hospital birth under the care of one or two midwives, take the chance to spend lots of time reviewing every part of your birth inclinations. Ideally, you chose these care providers from the start because they share your philosophy on birth. It still doesn't hurt to put your wishes in writing, so nothing is forgotten on the big day.

Birth Experience

An out-of-hospital birth plan may focus more on the specifics of the birth experience for you and your birth partners than on avoiding interventions.

Some items you might include are the desired ambiance of your birth location and the actions and the ideal approach of your birth team.

Transfer & Emergencies

Yet if you are preparing to give birth back home or in a birth center, there is even a little possibility that you or baby could end relocating to the hospital for some explanation. The best midwives have a transfer rate of about five percent. Nearly All of these moves are non-emergencies. In this argument, you should have a birth plan prepared that signifies your best birth in a worst-case scenario.

Even for a scheduled home birth or birth center delivery, you may create a birth plan that covers what might occur if you are transported to the hospital for any reason. Of course, you can't predict what that reason might be, so these preferences may change depending on what is possible at the time.

Sample Out of Hospital Birth Plan

Everyone's birth plan will be different, but here is an example of an actual natural home or birth center birth plan.

I would like it.

- Minimal noise or conversation
- Minimal lights
- No discussion of time
- Reassurance about the baby's well-being after fetal monitoring with the Doppler
- Encouragement and prayer
- Suggestions for more effective positions for laboring and pushing
- Recommendations and support during pushing to help prevent a tear
- To linger up until the cord stops pounding to cut
- To maintain as much skin-to-skin contact as possible, primarily if I do deliver in the tub
- Vitamin K to be administered orally
- No eye ointment to be administered
- The heel poke test to be done at a future checkup, but not on the day of birth
- Chlorhexidine wash during labor and antibiotics only after water breaks

Daddy, please remember to

- Cover or remove clocks and watches
- Remind me to empty my bladder every hour
- Make me eat throughout labor
- Make sure I get 4 ounces of liquid per hour
- Call for placenta encapsulation
- Have birth tub ready to return by home visit checkup

Here is an extensive list of considerations you may want to include in your birth plan.

First Stage Labor

Pain Relief

If you're planning a natural birth, obviously chemical pain relief is something you hope to avoid.

You will not want anyone around you who will pressure you just to go ahead and get an epidural, especially when you may be starting to like it yourself. Even the mere mention of drugs may throw off some moms' resolve. Ensure that everyone who will be at your birth is familiar with your goals for a natural delivery.

Many moms who give birth naturally find themselves asking for an epidural at some point during labor, whether at home or in the hospital. Have a plan for how you might like your birth partners or doula to respond in that situation.

Submersion in a warm water tub provides pain relief to many women. The added buoyancy of the water can also make it easier to assume and change labor positions. Although many hospitals have labor tubs available in some or all their rooms, most institutions and some care providers have policies against pushing and giving birth in water. However, no research shows the practice of water birth to increase risk. If you give birth at a birth center or home, having a water birth is almost always an option.

For most women in our culture, pain is a fact of giving birth, so you'll want to be able to maximize your options for natural pain relief, including using a variety of labor and pushing positions or laboring in the tub.

Freedom of Movement

Women's options for positions during the first and second stages are often limited for the convenience of care providers, whether it is ideal for getting the baby out most efficiently and safely. Most women in the US lay flat on their backs or in a semi-sitting position to push. It minimizes the opening of the pelvis and does not take advantage of gravity to assist in delivery. There are many more influential positions available to reduce the risk of forceps and vacuum-assisted delivery and concerns about the baby's heart rate. You will want to be free to assume any role your body is telling you during labor and pushing.

If you already know what positions you might like to try during labor, it might be a good idea to include them in your birth plan. This way, your birth partners or care providers will be able to prompt you if it seems like you need to try something different.

Fetal Monitoring

One of the medical interventions that can be most limiting to a woman's freedom of movement is fetal monitoring. Monitoring the baby's heart rate to make sure he is dealing with contractions well and is getting enough oxygen is essential. However, there are several options as to how it is accomplished.

In the hospital, external electronic fetal monitoring (EFM) can be done either intermittently or continuously. It requires the laboring mom to have the monitor strapped to her belly, thus limiting movement. There are some wireless devices available. EFM charts both the baby's heart rate and the strength of contractions.

The most invasive form of fetal monitoring is internal electronic fetal monitoring. It uses an electrode inserted into the baby's scalp and continuously monitors the baby's heart rate. Internal monitoring is used when severe distress is suspected. It requires that the bag of waters be broken and increases the risk of infection.

Electronic fetal monitoring is a widespread practice because it enables hospital staff to monitor multiple labors remotely, and it provides a record for potential lawsuits. EFM, whether continuous or intermittent, has not been shown to improve outcomes for mom and baby and increases the incidence of vacuum or forceps assisted delivery and c-section.

Instead, fetal monitoring may be done intermittently using a handheld Doppler ultrasound to listen to the baby's heartbeat. It is called "intermittent auscultation," and guidelines recommend monitoring for one minute every 15 to 30 minutes during the first stage and every 5 to 15 minutes during the second stage. This periodic monitoring allows you to continue to move around, walk, and it can even be used while you stay in the labor tub. If you are uncomfortable with your baby being exposed to ultrasound, a doctor or midwife can even use a fetoscope to check the heartbeat.

Birth Space, Relaxing space

Early on in your pregnancy, your midwife should talk to you about your options about where you would like to give birth to your baby. If this has not happened, you can request to go through it at your next appointment.

You can give birth at home or in a midwife-led unit (otherwise known as a 'birth center' or 'home from home') or in the central delivery unit (labor ward). Midwife-led companies may be freestanding (not attached to a hospital – though this is unlikely in the UK) or alongside (in the same building as the central labor ward – more usual).

It is well worth doing some research around each of the options below. After all, when you plan a holiday, chances are you spend at least a little (probably a lot!) of time researching your accommodation or the resort.

Or, if you were planning a wedding, you would likely spend a fair amount of time planning and looking into the venue and making sure it suited your needs.

So, take the time to research one of the biggest things you will ever do – have a baby.

Home Birth

Some women like the idea of giving birth at home – a place where they are in control and feel less like a patient, can have a bath, and eat and drink whatever and whenever they want. It is easier to distract yourself at home and carry on as usual for longer. You can book a home birth with your midwife. While you go into childbirth, you call your midwife, and she or a member of her team, who you likely will already know or have met, will come out to you at home. When the birth is imminent, she will usually call a second midwife to help her. If you book a home birth, you can change your mind at any time during your pregnancy, even during labor, and instead, opt to go to the birth center or labor ward.

What are the Benefits of a Home Birth?

If you plan a home birth, you are more likely to in advance have met the midwife who will take care of you during your labor (if your homebirth team offers what is called 'case loading' - where a named midwife will provide continuity of care). It can help you feel more comfortable and relaxed. Research has shown that labor usually progresses well at home when a woman knows her midwife.

You are in your domain, free to move as you wish, and eat and drink whatever you fancy whenever you fancy.

If you need to transfer to the hospital, your midwife will go with you. She may stay, or she may hand you over to the care of the hospital midwives on duty.

There is less pressure on labor within a particular timeframe, which means fewer interventions are offered to speed up your labor.

Should you require medical intervention, your midwife will arrange for you to go to your local hospital.

There is less risk of infection at a home birth.

You do get one-to-one care, as the midwife will be focusing on you and your baby, no one else. She will be regularly listening to your baby's heartbeat. She will not hesitate to suggest you transfer if she suspects a problem – something she will do long before any situation becomes an emergency.

Homebirth is strongly associated with improved breastfeeding outcomes.

Midwives are highly skilled and trained to deal with emergencies.

Homebirth and safety

Medical emergencies can occur anywhere, regardless of where a woman gives birth – but do remember that giving birth is generally very safe.

Midwives are highly skilled and trained to deal with any urgent situations while calling for further help. For example, if a post-partum hemorrhage were to happen, the midwife would have the initial drugs necessary to manage this and would arrange prompt transfer into the hospital.

In some cases, women requesting a home birth may be encouraged to give birth in the hospital, for example, in the event of a pregnancy lasting longer than 42 weeks, or the baby being in a breech position. Some women with less straightforward pregnancies or less usual factors to consider researching the pros and cons of their specific situation and make an informed decision to give birth at home still.

What's Available at a Home Birth?

You can have a water birth at home if you hire a pool. Sometimes you can find second-hand ones online and just buy a new liner. Your home birth team may have a pool you can hire.

You can hire or buy a TENS machine and use this.

You will have access to gas and air.

You may have access to either pethidine or diamorphine (opioids).

NICE guidance states that you should be supported and informed about your birthplace options. Your GP or midwife should not try to dissuade you from your choice unless they feel genuine medical reasons. If there is a medical reason why something is being suggested, then, of course, you'd be wise to discuss this and ask for sources of research and information on it. But the decision is always yours, and you are free to make your own choices even if your caregivers disagree with you.

Birth Centre

Sometimes a birth center is referred to as 'a home from home,' or 'midwife-led suite.' Giving birth in a birth center can be an excellent option for many women who have had straightforward pregnancies. Birth centers are run by midwives and do not routinely use medical interventions if labor progresses well. As many labors go well, birth centers are an excellent alternative to giving birth in the hospital.

Should a woman require any medical intervention, she can transfer to the labor ward. Most birth centers are in the same building, even on the same floor, as the central hospital/labor ward, which many women find reassuring.

Pros of Using a Birth Centre

Birth centers feel more homely and less clinical, which in turn can make you feel more relaxed.

They are often more spacious, with more equipment available, such as birthing stools, birth balls, and padded floors to comfortably kneel on.

They may have a double bed available for after the birth for your birth partner to stay overnight, but this is sometimes tucked out of the way or folded up against the wall to encourage women not to hop up on it! Research shows that being upright and mobile during active labor has many benefits, shortening labor and making it feel more manageable.

Birth centers' birth is seen as a regular event rather than a risky one, and having a straightforward delivery is much more likely. Exact birth means giving birth vaginally, without any procedures or interventions such as assisted birth (forceps or ventose), induction of labor, or cesarean birth.

Some centers allow you to stay in the room, with your partner and baby, for your whole stay, though you will need to transfer out if someone wants to use the space. Others request that you transfer to the postnatal ward at some point after the birth.

The midwives who work in a birth center have often chosen this environment as they have a passionate interest in supporting women to birth with little or no intervention.

Cons of Using a Birth Centre

If you decide you want an epidural, you need to transfer to the labor ward. If your birth center is not located within the hospital, ask your midwife which unit you would move to and how long this would take.

What's Available at a Birth Centre?

Very often, pools are plumbed in, or inflatable ones are available.

You will have access to Entonox (gas and air).

Sometimes the midwives are trained in and can offer aromatherapy massage or reflexology.

Often you will be able to have pethidine or diamorphine for pain relief during labor should you want this.

There is less equipment visible, which helps to give a feel of birth being a normal event.

If your baby needed special care, they would be transferred to the special care baby unit, which in most cases, will be in the same building.

While the transfer may not happen instantly unless it is an emergency, you can always change your mind. If you want to transfer out of the birth center and onto the labor ward, you wish to – for example, if you decided you now wanted an epidural (epidurals are not available on the birth center).

Hospital Birth/Labor Ward

Some women choose to give birth to the labor ward as they find it reassuring.

If a woman has consultant-led care, she may be more likely to be offered the labor ward than the birth center.

However, being in the hospital environment makes it more likely that you will be offered interventions, which is something to bear in mind. There is also less privacy in a hospital setting.

If you have had a complicated pregnancy or are likely to require a cesarean birth for medical reasons, you will be encouraged to give birth in the hospital, in the labor ward.

Midwives will still provide your care, but doctors will be available if required. It is unlikely that you will have met your midwife in advance of your birth.

What is Available on the Labor Ward?

You will have access to an epidural, pethidine/diamorphine, and Entonox (gas and air).

Some labor wards have birthing pools available – ask your midwife or check the Which? Birth website to see if bringing your pool in is an option.

Access to a special care baby unit.

Some women like to start in the birth center and transfer to the labor ward if they feel like an epidural. Once you are in your room in the labor ward, you can make it your own. You may like to:

- Dim the lights as low as you can.
- Cover windows with blackout blinds.
- Bring battery-operated fairy lights for a beautiful, soft glow.
- Cover any unused equipment with a scarf or blanket/towel to make it feel less clinical.
- Birth balls should be provided, but you can bring your own.
- Raise or lower the bed. So, you are not tempted to get on it and not move around much after that.
- Bring music.
- Bring an essential oil of your choice to breathe in from a piece of fabric.
- Cover the clock, so you are not focused on it.

Turning a Birth Partner into Hypnobirthing Partner

During pregnancy, your partner often feels like a bystander. Partners (many of whom have played a crucial role at the beginning) are now left to watch you blossom and grow, without ever really being able to understand or feel what you are experiencing. Many partners will often leave the finding out about birth and baby matters to the mum and will only attend an antenatal class if they are asked to.

Unlike many mainstream antenatal classes, a hypnobirthing course is about connecting both parents with the pregnancy, labor, and birth (and if your birth partner isn't the baby's father, it is highly recommended that whoever you choose attends the course with you). Your birth partner needs to understand all the aspects of a hypnobirthing course along with you so that they can fully support you when the big day arrives.

By attending a hypnobirthing course with you, your birth partner is thoroughly involved in the experience.

They can be hands-on during the course and will learn to:

- understand the process of labor
- understand, explore, and follow your birth preferences
- ask the right questions for your circumstances
- read the hypnobirthing scripts to you for maximum effect
- appropriately, calmly, and confidently support you during labor
- look after your newborn baby

You can now see it is essential for birth partners to take part in your hypnobirthing journey / Program for mums to feel 100% supported.

There are so many advantages to your birth partner attending a course with you – most notably, that the experience of labor and birth is not unfamiliar when the time comes.

Your birth partner is one of the most influential people involved in your birth. It's essential to have someone there in whom you have total confidence and who can support you 100%. Your birth partner must be very clear about your hopes, feelings, and preferences for the birth so that he or she can speak up and advocate for you if needed.

In most cases, the baby's father will be the lucky one who gets to share this exceptional moment. Still, you may also opt for your closest friend, your mother, another member of the family, or a doula, as well as or instead of him or her. Indeed, you may feel that you would like more than one person with you during labor and birth. If so, explain your reasons to your birth partner about having someone else there, saying that they could give him or her support too. The crucial thing is that you choose someone (or people) that you completely trust and with whom you are at ease. They must be a rock for you, should the going got tough. It is also a good idea to organize a back-up if, for some reason, your first choice is absent. Most close friends and relatives will jump at the opportunity of helping you and witnessing a birth.

The birth partner's job is a significant one. It's not just about providing a hand to squeeze or being able to pant loudly with you, as TV or films sometimes portray! The primary responsibility he or she will have been to offer you complete support and encouragement and keep you as comfortable as possible during labor and birth. You need someone prepared to respond to your every whim on the big day, and not be annoyed when you change your mind and just want the room to be silent for hours on end.

This person must be happy to pace the room with you, or to help you with optimal positioning, or to massage you just like you learned in your hypnobirthing preparation. It should be someone who won't be insulted if you get grouchy or suddenly ask to be left alone, and someone who will remain strong during difficult moments, should they arise. Lastly, it has to be someone who can be your voice: represent your thoughts and feelings, and stand up for what you want or need, if, during labor, you are unable to (or would rather not) do so yourself.

Your birth partner will experience the whole unique process. They will be the first to see your baby's head emerging into the world (if they choose to look) and will get the chance to cut the umbilical cord if they fancy it. It may also be their role to remain with your baby if you need medical attention or feel tired after birth, or if, for any reason, the baby needs assistance. Your birth partner may have to endure quite a lot during labor and delivery, but in doing so, you will receive the greatest reward: they will have the honor of being one of the first people to get a precious cuddle.

For them to be fully aligned with your thinking and know precisely what you are likely to need during labor and birth, it is highly recommended that they do the entire hypnobirthing course with you. Not only will it be more informed about late pregnancy, labor, and birth, but together you will discuss your preferences and make decisions that feel right for both of you and your baby, beforehand and on the day. Of course, they will also learn how best to support you during labor, physically as well as emotionally, so that you can focus on connecting with your mind, body, and baby.

'A hypnobirthing course is a wonderful experience. When preparing for your baby there is so much to think about. Learning the relaxation scripts and doing them with my wife helped me to understand the level of relaxation that she needs to be feeling. It was informative and fun.' Mayank, father-to-be.

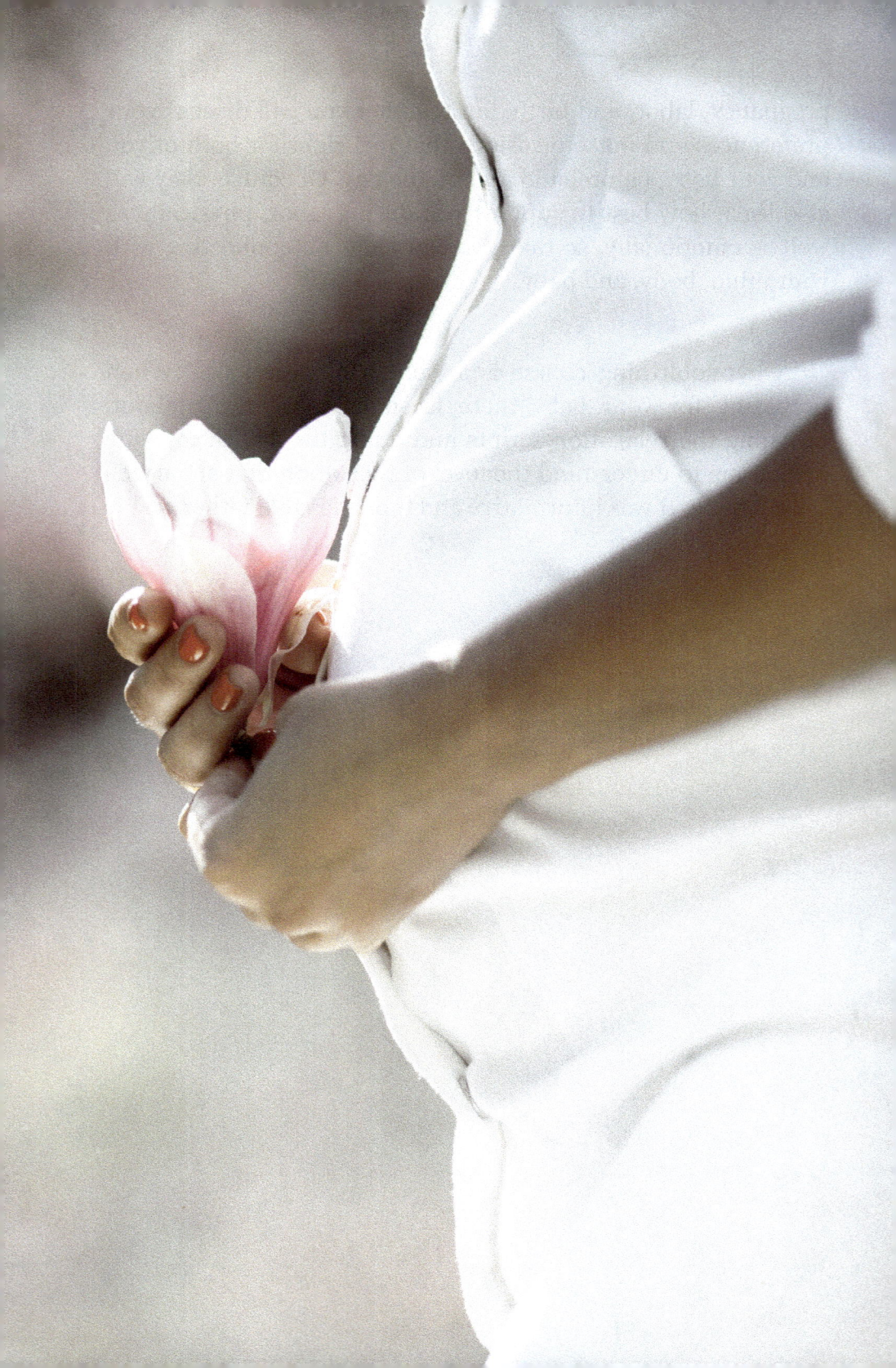

Chapter 13: When will birth begin?

Weeks or days, before the labor begins, your body gradually prepares for birth, and you may also notice a difference in the way you feel. There is likely to be an emphatic 'nesting instinct as you prepare for life with your new baby and a need to focus your attention on taking care of yourself. Hormonal secretions increase currently to initiate the first physical changes in your body and to prepare you emotionally for the intensity of the birth experience.

Waves of energy may alternate with a need to rest and sleep. Try to surrender to these rhythms and to go along with what your body tells you. You will transition into labor more quickly if you simplify your daily activities and rest whenever needed. Allow yourself to 'space out' and get onto the same wavelength as your baby.

When you feel like being active, carry on with basic household tasks, spending some time every day in the open air, practicing some simple yoga, meditation, and breathing, or having a relaxing massage. Getting into a swimming pool will relieve you from the heaviness of the weight you are carrying and help you to sleep better. If you have a home birth, you might enjoy a trial run of setting up and filling your pool and relaxing in the water for a while or spend more time relaxing and meditating in the bath.

'It was wonderful to use the pool in the last days of my

pregnancy, not only because it made the 'bump' less bulky, but also because it gave me relief from the hot weather we were experiencing at the time.'

Don't worry if your sleep patterns become very erratic and unusual – it's good practice for night-time parenting. Your dreams may also be more vivid. If you are resting a lot and getting some gentle exercise, your body will make sure that you sleep when you need to. If you have an active toddler or other children to look after, this is a critical time to be together before the arrival of the new baby. It's wise to arrange some daily childcare too, so you can also have enough time alone to rest and relax.

You may experience a lot of emotions from excitement to terror. At times you may feel vulnerable and experience some anxiety about what is about to happen to you. In this case, taking the homeopathic remedy, aconite may be helpful. You may also feel blissfully contented and peaceful. Some women positively glow with radiant energy as the pregnancy reaches full bloom.

It is an excellent time to consider taking a supplement of evening primrose oil, which is beneficial in ripening the cervix (see below). You can consume one 500mg capsule three times a day from 36 weeks until birth. You can also drink three cups of organic raspberry leaf tea daily throughout this period.

It is a mild uterine tonic and stimulant with proven beneficial effects on the uterus. These supplements to your diet will support your body's natural preparation for birth and help to ensure that labor starts on time.

Pre-Labor

Runs of frequent or mild contractions, which usually feel a bit like period pains, may stop and start over several days. Unusual lower back pain or a feeling of being disconnected or extra sensitive are also possible. The build-up to labor begins long before it starts. You may not even notice it but there are changes that are happening.

Diarrhea is expected as the bowel empties in readiness for birth, increasing mucous discharge from the vagina. The practice contractions you will have felt throughout pregnancy will now increase in frequency and intensity. These contractions do the critical work of preparing the cervix for dilation. It is the ring of muscular tissue at the base of the uterus that forms the opening to the womb. Situated at the top of the vagina, the cervix is closed in pregnancy and sealed with a plug of thick mucus.

During the final weeks of pregnancy, hormones secreted within the cervix itself cause it to soften – or 'ripen' – in readiness to open during labor. The action from the contractions gradually draws up the muscular fibers of the cervix so that it 'effaces' or becomes much thinner. By the time labor starts, it will thin from its standard thickness of about 3 cm to the thinness of a sheet of paper. It may even open a centimeter or two – but this is not yet established labor. The cervix is usually tucked quite far back in the pelvic cavity, and it will move forward to the center of the lower uterus during this phase. These crucial changes of pre-labor generally go unnoticed. However, some women are susceptible to pre-labor contractions. Although they are relatively mild in intensity, they can keep you awake at night. If this happens, resting and sleeping whenever activity stops or slows down is essential to conserve your energy.

Alternatively, it can be comfortable to lie resting forwards in a kneeling position supported on a beanbag or a big pile of cushions on the bed. Ensure that you eat small, easily digestible meals at frequent intervals and drink plenty of clear fluids.

The massive increase in hormones currently also further softens the ligaments that bind the pelvic joints, preparing the bony passage to open to its widest for your baby to descend and pass through during the birth. The pelvic floor muscles form a 'hammock' through which the urethra, vagina, and anus open. Hormones also soften these ligaments. It is to allow them to stretch and open as the baby passes through during birth.

The Show

As pre-labor contractions thin the cervix, the jelly-like mucous plug that seals the cervix may be expelled. It is called having a 'show.' This may appear blood-stained and red, pink, or brown and may be quite thick and glue-like in texture or thinner and more liquid. It can come away gradually a little at a time, or all at once. A show may occur sometime in the week or so before labor starts, immediately before established labor begins or further on in labor. Don't panic if you see a show – there is probably some time to go before you are really in labor.

Waters Breaking

Inside the uterus, your baby floats in the amniotic fluid, surrounded by the strong double membrane of the amniotic sac. In about 20 percent of pregnancies, the first sign that labor is imminent is the natural rupture of these membranes. It releases part or most of the amniotic fluid and is called the breaking of the waters. More amniotic fluid is produced throughout labor – so this does not mean 'dry' labor. The sudden drop in pressure within the uterus may trigger the onset of labor contractions immediately or within an hour or so. The waters can also break much later once labor has already started. Frequently this happens just before or even as the baby is being born. Occasionally the membranes remain intact, and the baby is born 'in a caul.' In this case, the midwife will rupture the membranes as the baby emerges.

However, it's also common for membranes to rupture a day or two before labor starts. It marginally increases the risk of infection, since the protective barrier formed by the membranes is gone. While the condition is highly unlikely, you may come under considerable pressure to induce labor if your membranes rupture early. The risk of disease does marginally increase over time and how long you can wait is something you need to discuss with your midwife. However, labor will usually start spontaneously within 48 hours, and most practitioners can be persuaded to stay that long. Beyond this, most midwifery guidelines will rule out water labor and birth or home birth, and induction is likely recommended. Common-sense precautions to prevent infection are to stay close to home where you are naturally immune to the household bacteria, to avoid intercourse or introducing anything into the vagina, avoiding lying in the bath or the birth pool, and to wash after emptying bladder or bowel. If there is no sign of contractions after 24 hours, it may also help take a high dose vitamin C supplement once a day and garlic capsules three times a day to prevent infection. In the improbable event of an illness, you would notice an unpleasant odor and probably have a temperature. In this case, a cesarean would be necessary.

Your Baby Before Birth

While your body prepares itself for labor, your baby is getting ready to leave the womb. In the final weeks before the birth, the journey downwards begins as the baby's head 'engages' or enters the pelvic brim. In some pregnancies, especially second or subsequent ones, engagement may not happen until labor starts.

As described, when your baby is ready to breathe independently, hormonal secretions from the baby's lungs will initiate labor. This stimulus combines with that created by an increase in pressure. It is on the base of the uterus from the baby's head, as it descends more in-depth into the pelvis to initiate the start of labor. Some babies remain active throughout pre-labor, while others seem to Move Much Less, As Though They Have An Ample Rest Or Sleep, Getting Ready For The Birth.

Approaching Your Due Date

Sometimes nothing much unusual seems to be happening as the due date comes and goes, and you may well be wondering if pre-labor is ever going to start.

Jacqueline Vincent Priya, in her book Birth Traditions and Modern Pregnancy Care, says: 'When I talked to pregnant women from traditional societies, their happy vagueness about when the birth was likely to take place always amused me. After my own experiences with modern doctors who provided a specific 'B-day' and started to worry if the baby hadn't arrived by that date, the relaxed attitude of these women was a tonic. They usually knew within a month or to when the baby night comes and trusted their internal knowledge and experience of the pregnancy as to when the birth would take place.'

She describes some of the unique rituals used traditionally to ensure that the mother goes into labor relaxed and confident. It seems a very long way indeed from the experiences of pregnant women who are under pressure to start labor 'on time' in our culture. Stress, anxiety, and worry are counterproductive to the hormone secretion everyone is waiting for – so try to keep up your faith in your body and trust its wisdom.

The Tyranny Of The Due Date

One can be disheartened to find that you are still pregnant a week or more beyond this date, even more so if you are told that using a birth pool is no longer possible. The hospital is talking about booking date to induce labor. Unnecessary inductions are the cause of many complications in delivery. Since most women go beyond their due date, this is an issue for many women planning to use a birth pool. The information will help to guide you if you find yourself 'overdue.'

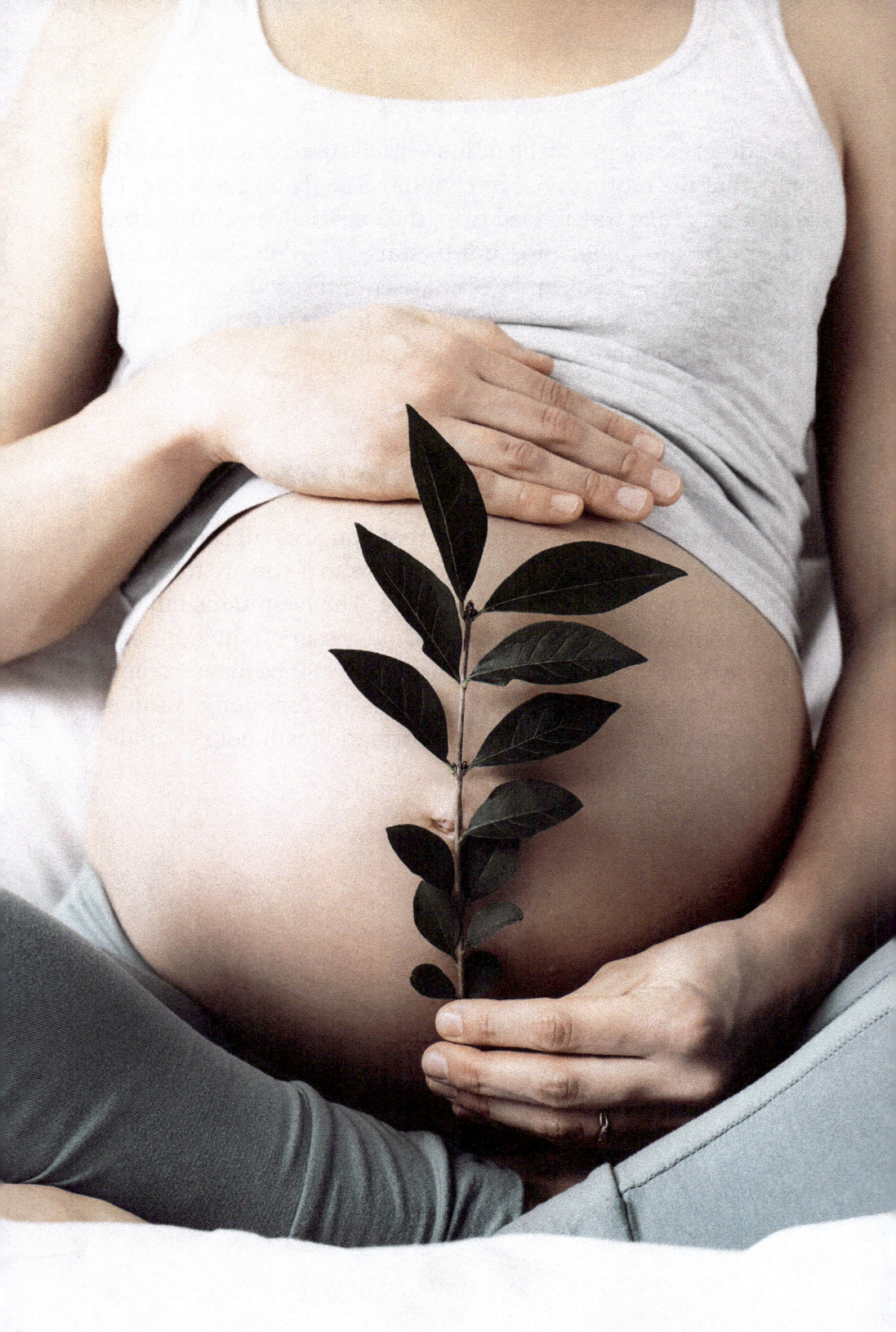

Chapter 14: The Birth

Labor is usually divided into three main stages. Here is an overview of each step, and how you can use the Blissful Birth techniques at each stage.

First Stage

The first stage of labor is where your body is preparing to give birth. Your contractions will help to thin out and open your cervix ready for the Second Stage. It begins when your contractions start and end when your cervix is fully dilated to around 10cm.

The first stage is often sub-divided into two or three phases:

Early Labor

Early labor starts when you begin to get regular contractions. At this stage, it can sometimes be hard to know you are in labor. It is because the contractions are usually quite far apart and relatively short - typically coming every 10-20 minutes and lasting around 30 seconds - so many women confuse them as Braxton-Hicks practice contractions.

Early labor is usually comfortable and makes up the bulk

of your birth experience, so it will give you plenty of time to mentally prepare, make any final arrangements, and get some rest. Your cervix will begin dilating up to around 5cm during this phase.

Some women get a strong urge to 'nest' in early labor - I know I did - and doing any outstanding housework not only helps you pass the time and gives you some gentle exercise to help things along but can also help put your mind at ease that everything is ready at home.

It is an ideal time to reinforce your relaxation anchor, to listen to the birth rehearsal or favorite place MP3's again, take a gentle walk (which helps things along) or just chill out and relax.

Remember, your body needs water so that your muscles can work effectively, so make sure you stay well hydrated by drinking plenty of water and empty your bladder frequently.

Active Labor

As the first stage of labor continues, your contractions will gradually get closer together, last longer, and become more intense. When your contractions are around 3-5 minutes apart and lasting up to a minute, this is often known as active labor.

When you get to this stage, you'll probably find your contractions harder to ignore. Activities such as walking or sitting on the toilet can often feel good, as can massage, or a warm bath or shower. Your cervix will continue dilating from around 5 to 8cm during this phase.

Now is the time that you'll probably want your birth partner to start helping you use favorite relaxation and self-hypnosis techniques and coaching you to breathe through contractions.

You might also want to play the Relaxation MP3 at this stage, as it contains binaural beats to help you stay deeply relaxed.

With each contraction, prompt yourself that you are moving one step closer to meeting your baby and take a moment to imagine that moment in detail when you hold your baby in your arms for the first time.

If the mother is thinking of giving birth in a hospital or birthing center, you'll be calling in to let them know your progress and going in at some point during active labor. Similarly, if you give birth at home, you'll contact the midwife to let her know you are in active labor. There is no such perfect timing to go in - you'll know when it is the right time for you.

Transition

The final and shortest phase of First Stage labor is known as transition, and this is where your body is finishing the dilation of your cervix and getting ready to switch to the downward, baby delivering muscles.

Contractions, in this phase, can come every 2-3 minutes and last around 60-90 seconds. You'll probably start to feel the urge to push, as your baby will be moving into the final position for stage two. Your cervix will also complete its dilation from around 8 to 10 cm during this last phase of First Stage labor.

Most women automatically and naturally go into hypnosis during this phase - even if they have never practiced self-hypnosis! It is because hypnosis is one of your body's natural protection mechanisms and is the body's way of helping you move through this phase.

Because of this, some women report feeling 'foggy' during this phase - and many women experience a time distortion (a classic sign of hypnosis), which makes this phase seem to go so much more quickly.

All the Blissful Birth work you have done so far will help your transition be a very positive experience. During this phase, you will be especially sensitive to the suggestions of others. If you remember the Blissful Birth report, this is where I was convinced to deliver on my back! So, your birth partner and caregivers can help you by giving you positive, encouraging suggestions.

Second Stage: Pushing

The first stage of labor ends when your cervix is fully dilated. Unlike transition, your contractions in the second stage will probably ease up and start coming a little further apart again, giving you a chance to rest in between.

As this stage progresses, you'll start getting the overwhelming urge to push. The pushing sensation is very much like the urge to empty your bowels, and if you are pushing right, chances are you will poo a little.

Let's set the record straight here. Pretty much every woman giving birth does this, and midwives are expecting it - if you are pushing right and there is anything left up there, it will come out! It is nature's way of achieving sure not anything gets in the form of the birth process.

Most women describe this stage as the most empowering. You'll know the end is in sight, and each contraction brings you a step closer to meeting your baby. If you are using an upright birth position, gravity will also help your baby keep coming down, rather than the 'two steps forward, one step back' which can happen if you are giving birth on your back.

By only pushing when you feel the healthy, natural urge, rather than when anyone else tells you to, you can help avoid any tearing and even the infamous 'ring of fire.'

Breathing is the key to this stage. Make sure you push each breathes down to your abdomen as this not only helps keep you relaxed but makes sure you get plenty of oxygen to your muscles. Your midwife may tell you to stop pushing as your baby's head crowns so she can check the cord position - you will find 'candle blowing' an effective way to overcome the urge.

The second stage ends with the birth of your baby! Congratulations!

Third Stage: Delivering the Placenta

Shortly after delivery, usually within an hour, your uterus will begin to contract again, which helps separate the placenta ready to be delivered. When your midwife sees that separation is complete, she may ask you to push to help the placenta gently. It is usually one short easy push that's comfortable.

Hospitals routinely offer an injection to speed up the placenta (known as an "assisted third stage"). It can make the third stage much shorter and reduce blood loss. However, it requires the early clamping of the umbilical cord.

Positions for Giving Birth

The positions that you choose during labor are essential, as you need to feel comfortable but also in control and support.

Most women think about lying on their backs to give birth, which is the typical image portrayed in the media. It is also the preferred position in many hospitals as it is more convenient for the midwives/medical team to gain access and manage the delivery.

However, lying down has many disadvantages. Firstly, it can restrict your pelvis' ability to open by around 30%. It can also slow the contractions down, makes it is difficult to move around, and it puts more significant pressure on the perineum. It can all lead to the need for forceps or ventose delivery and increase the chance of tearing. It also does not allow gravity to aid delivery.

However, if you give birth in an upright position, the combination of the contractions, pushing, and the force of gravity is a powerful one. Several studies have reported that women giving birth upright tend to experience less pain during and after delivery, whereas those lying down experienced more pain and less comfort.

Some of the common positions used for giving birth are

Squatting

Squatting down helps to open the pelvis and makes pushing through your contractions more effective. It uses gravity; however, it is a difficult position to stay in for any length of time and makes it difficult to move to a resting position

Kneeling/Leaning

You are kneeling either on the bed or a pile of cushions on the floor. You may also be leaning forward onto a birthing ball. It is particularly suitable for strong contractions as you can rock backward and forwards or bear down, without putting too much pressure on the legs. It uses gravity and can be less tiring than squatting.

I used this position for the birth of my second son, who arrived in 17 minutes! What I liked about this position was that my birth partner, Rob, could kneel the other side of the birthing ball, hold my hands during contractions, reassure me, and keep my hair out of my face!

All Fours

Kneeling on all fours is a good position for a large baby, and it can also assist with the rotation of a posterior presentation. It can slow the contractions, but this can be good if you need a break. It can also be an excellent position to deliver the head as movement is slower, and the risk of tearing is reduced. Gravity is not as sufficient, but as the weight is taken away from your spine, it is useful if you are experiencing back pain.

Sitting

Sitting and semi-sitting are comfortable positions to adopt in a hospital bed. It can be quite relaxing and makes it easy to rest between contractions. It has some benefit of gravity, but the disadvantage is that you are sitting on your coccyx (tailbone), so movement is reduced, making it harder for the baby to descend. There is also some stress on the perineum but not as much as when lying.

Lying

Lying down does not make use of gravity, so it can be an excellent position to help slow a baby who is coming too fast. The advantage of this is that it can give the perineum more time to stretch naturally, therefore avoiding a tear. The disadvantage of lying down is that without the help of gravity, it can make pushing longer.

Note - As with all decisions regarding birth, it is essential to adopt positions that you feel comfortable physically and emotionally. There is no right or wrong - everything has advantages and disadvantages, but ultimately, it is your choice.

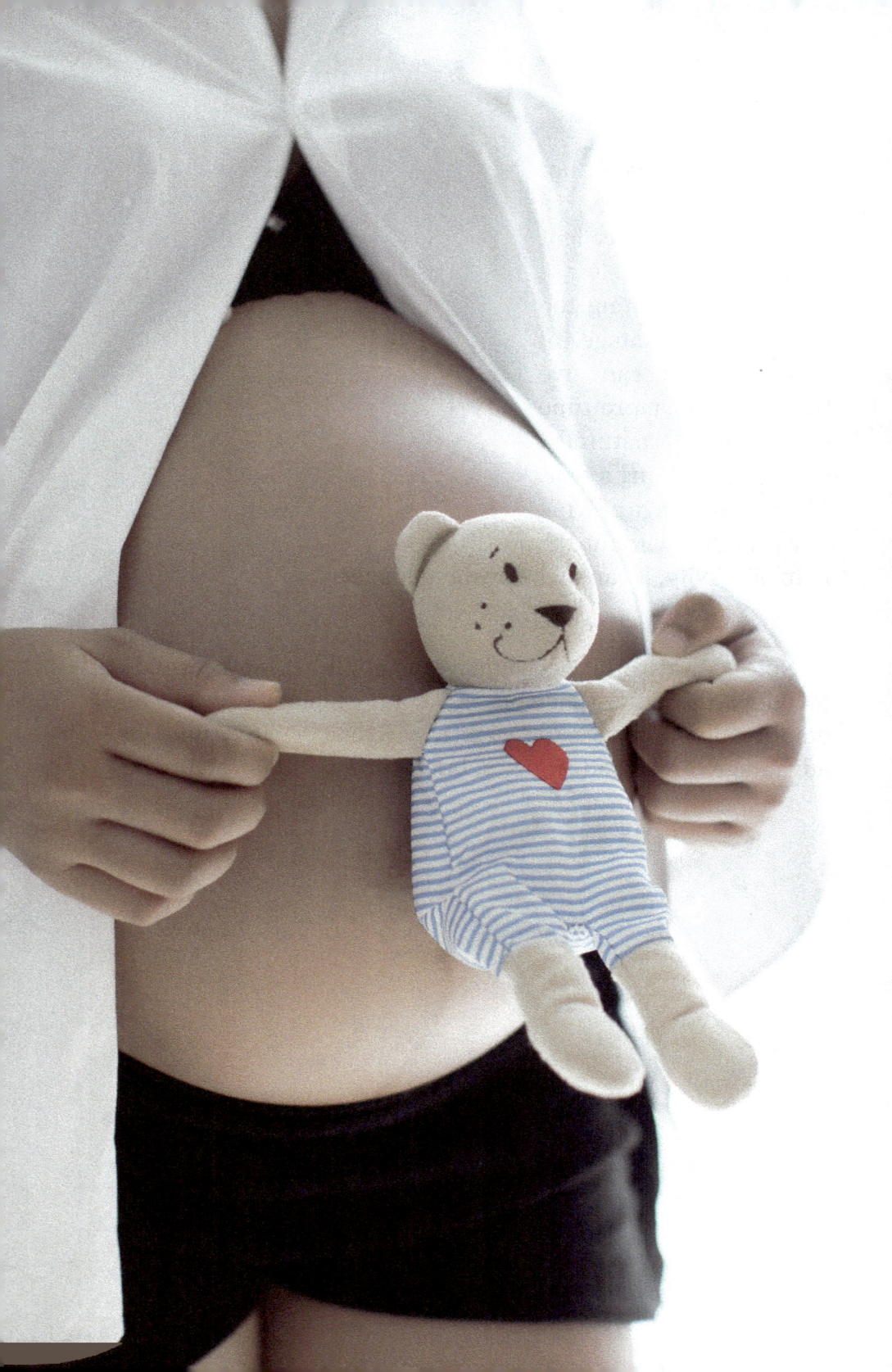

Chapter 15: The Umbilical Code

Until very recently, we assumed that the environment in the uterus was dark, warm, and silent, much like a cave in the deep bowels of Earth. The child in the womb was separate from the outside world, it was believed, and that world did not penetrate the protective surroundings of the amniotic sac and the mother's skin and tissue.

Recent studies have revealed that this assumption is wrong and that the intrauterine world of the child is subject to changes caused by both the own unborn growth and the actions in the world outside the mother's body. Other research has shown that all human senses are working to some degree by the time the unborn is in the second trimester of development. Tests have shown that the unborn will respond to pressure, touch, heat, movement, sound, pain, and even certain types of taste.

Your unborn's environment shifts with the stimuli—including sights, odors, sounds, tastes, and touch—that you experience during pregnancy. Unborn contribute to this environment themselves, shifting in the womb, "playing" with their fingers or bodies and pushing with arms, legs, or head. The amniotic fluid changes during pregnancy, too. Depending on your diet and the release of hormones in your body, the fluid's chemical makeup alters. During the last trimester, the unborn may swallow and excrete this fluid, again changing the composition of his environment.

Do perceptions experienced regularly during pregnancy, even before the brain develops, affect the cell development of the body, which in turn perhaps affects the structure of the emerging brain? These are essential considerations for deciding how to care for yourself while creating a new life and a world for your baby.

So, we can ask ourselves: How does the emotion of the mother communicate with the unborn? How does it influence the development of the body/brain/mind? and the adapting skills of the infant? How can and does the brain/mind of the unborn integrate the experience of the mother in a way that begins to shape a healthy, well-adapted, well-bonded infant?

Nature Versus Nurture

The correct environment is necessary to bring out the best and diminish the worst in the constitution and personality of a child's genetic makeup. The proper intrauterine environment and mother–father–child extrauterine interaction is necessary. It is to enhance the best of a child's temperament and to contain the worst. A basic genetic makeup appears to be neither good nor bad; it just is. What is important is the effectiveness or ineffectiveness of the child's developmental environment concerning her basic personality.

Even during pregnancy, be aware of the needs of not only you and your unborn but also any other children you may have. Keep in mind that these needs change and that each child is different, even in the womb. What is suitable for one child may not be healthy for another. When you realize and implement this, it could create havoc in a household. One child might ask, for example, "Why do I have to go to bed earlier? I'm older," or

"Why can't I run and jump for more than fifteen minutes? Why do you pay the babysitter to take Karen outside to encourage her to run and jump?"

As the socialist philosophy goes, "each according to his needs" or, in the vernacular, "different strokes for different folks." The question is knowing what is right for each mother-infant dyad and following through on the proper schedule, balanced diet, nursing style, and so on. All babies need structure and respect, but some need more structure; some require you to listen more.

All is potentiality: genes, metabolism, personality traits. It is the environment that creates the actualization and the proper balance of infinite possibilities. As parents, we cannot relinquish responsibility to genetics. We must take charge and make the right environmental influences.

But do we need more responsibility and something else to feel guilty about? Just when we women are finally out there in the workforce, science tells us how very, very important our role as mothers is. To prevent violence, we need to address it before its onset. The best money the government could spend to avoid future violence would be to create free prenatal development education centers and to pay mothers to breastfeed.

To gain some insight, we might look at the laboratory research, where psych biologist Robert Cairns has given us vital information about aggressive behavior in mice. When a genetically aggressive mouse is overreactive and edgy, Dr. Cairns reports, another mouse in contact with it can influence the aggressor so that it backs off rather than making an all-out attack. The second mouse, the nonaggressive mouse, accomplishes this change by freezing motion and not responding to the aggressor. Dr. Cairns states, "It's not a gene or a biochemical ... behaving but an integrated organism behaving within a real world."

In other words, neither the genetic makeup nor the history of the mouse is stopping its aggression. At least in part, its actions are determined by the response it has received. Dr. Cairns continues, "On the interim of the organism, the success or failure of behavioral accommodation in reducing the threat and promoting well-being is recorded in the language of neurochemistry and hormones."

Breastfeeding is social interaction at a primal level. If our actions, like the mouse's, have a large behavioral component, you might say that breastfeeding is the mother's lab of gene/environmental interaction. The World Health Organization stresses, for example, that every child should be breastfed until six months of age, as part of the environment she is born into. Here you can observe your baby's interaction with the mother and mother's interaction with the baby. What do you need to be in balance? What does your infant need, and how can you both be in harmony together? Where do you need to shift so he can shift comfortably? What escalates undesirable behavior, and what diminishes it? Just as with the mouse, the social behavior of your infant. It is continually growing as it relates to you and your actions.

The structure of the brain is formed by interpersonal experience. As a product of brain activity, the mind emerges. Of concern in this process is how the mother's experiences while pregnant and her perception of her past experiences affect the physical, emotional, and behavioral development of the unborn. Is there an umbilical code, an interpersonal relationship between the mother and her developing child that announces how a particular mind/body interaction of the mother affects the specific areas of the brain/mind/body of the unborn and his subsequent interaction with the world?

Each of us is genetically programmed, but what is it that organizes that material in us individually? Various experiences and energy in the form of biochemical messages flow between mother and infant. How do these experiences and perceptions translate and perhaps transform the nervous system of the unborn? Perhaps each mother is not only growing a body/brain but also creating the mind of her unborn.

Although we don't know how, exactly, we know that when the unborn's brain is developing, the mother participates in the activation of neurons or electrical activity in the brain. The flow of energy in the mother's brain affects the flow of energy in her unborn's brain. In the fourth week of gestation, your unborn's cranial nerve motor neurons are forming. These control the muscles of the eye lens, throat, and tongue.

Amazingly, this can occur even before a mother knows she is pregnant. The stem of the brain and your unborn's ears are simultaneously developing. At what crucial time in development are the mental processes of the unborn being established? We learn through our senses and perceive through our senses.

It is conceivable that each of the mother's sensory perceptions interacts with fetal development. Still, it is also probable that the interaction of the senses establishes a pattern of neural firing. Imagine, for example, that a mother is driving along in Malibu and passes the septic tanks there, with their intermittent lousy odor. This smell could lead to a particular neural firing if paired with a memory such as Frank McCourt describes in his book *Angela's Ashes* of growing up poor in Ireland near the public toilet. The smell could mean something different, however, depending on the mother's thoughts at the time. She might instead think, "Oh! I'm halfway home. Look at the waves; they're perfect. In twenty minutes, I'll be in my wetsuit surfing. Isn't it funny how we all put up with the periodic stench of Malibu just to live here in such incredible beauty?"

As you can see, these are very different thought patterns, and very different neural firings could take place. How would each affect the neural release of the mother and her unborn? Even before the brain develops, these perceptions, experienced regularly during pregnancy, may affect the cell development of the fetal body, which in turn perhaps affects the structure of the emerging brain.

Chapter 16: Have a Green and Gorgeous Pregnancy

Your body will go beyond enormous physical modifications over the next nine months, so this is the perfect time to indulge in a beauty routine that makes you feel gorgeous inside and out. But you must be cautious; several of the products on store shelves that claim to make you beautiful may be harmful to you, your baby, and the planet. Use the tips to pamper yourself with an eco-savvy style.

Green Beauty Basics

Over the next nine months, every inch of your body will change in one way or another. As your body expands to adjust to your growing baby, you may notice differences in your skin, hair, and even your fingernails. And at a time when you may be feeling most self-conscious about your body, it can be easy to fall prey to the constant bombardment from the global cosmetics industry as it aims to sell you products that claim to make you look younger, thinner, and more gorgeous.

Unfortunately, many conventional beauty products contain ingredients that are harmful to human and environmental health. You might think that if they are on the store shelves, they must be safe, but there is minimal oversight over the safety of products from the personal care industry.

More than 1,110 personal-product ingredients have been

banned for use in cosmetics in the European Union because of concerns that they may cause cancer, congenital disabilities, or reproductive disorders. By contrast, only ten are banned in the United States.

Agreeing to the Environmental Working Group: 89 percent of the 10,500 ingredients used in personal care products have not been evaluated for safety by the FDA. It is the agency that regulates the personal care product industry. Even the Cosmetic Ingredient Review, an in-house panel appointed by the cosmetics industry, has not evaluated it or by anyone else.

Remember that every personal care product you use in your beauty regimen, whether it is soap or mascara, will eventually wash off of your body and into the environment, where its presence may affect plants, birds, fish, and other wildlife.

Does this mean that you must go without washing your hair or applying cosmetics to be green? Certainly not! Fortunately, it is easy to green your beauty regimen if you know what to look for. Here's how to enjoy a green and gorgeous pregnancy.

Use a Little Less

Now that you have a baby on board, it may be time to reevaluate just how many beauty products you use each day. Sure, cosmetic companies want you to think that you need every lotion and potion on the store shelves to look beautiful, but you will find that when you use clean, all-natural beauty products, you only need the basics to look and feel your best. All the rest is a waste of money—a waste of energy and resources for the planet.

Also, be conscious of the amount of each product that you use each day. Do you consistently squeeze a massive dollop of styling products into your hand only to wash most of it away? Try to use a little less of each of your beauty products to make them go further. It will save you money and minimize the number of chemicals that eventually wash down the drain.

Be Kind to Animals

You don't have to be a vegetarian to realize that animal testing is needless, wrong, and just plain brutal. Watch for products branded with the Leaping Bunny. This symbol, created by the Coalition for Consumer Information on Cosmetics (www.leapingbunny.org), is the only international standard label for personal care products indicating that they are brutality-free, and they have not been tested on animals.

In the past, manufacturers had to choose between minimal safety testing of their products and safety testing that used animals. But now, scientists can use cultures of human skin cells and tissues to test the reaction and absorption rate of chemicals, or a combination of chemicals, on the skin.

Go Oil-Free

You probably already know that the consumption of fossil fuels is not so great for the planet. But you may not realize that petroleum is also used for a few products in your bathroom vanity. Petroleum derivates may be found in personal care products such as lip balm, lotions, and lubricants, as well as the plastics used in sanitary products.

Avoid Aerosols

The chemicals applied in aerosols are no longer a threat to the ozone layer. Still, these chemicals have been replaced with petroleum propellants whose production creates the greenhouse gases that lead to global warming. Choose no aerosol or pump-style products for your personal care routine.

Skip the Chemical Cocktail

There are a few questionable chemical components such as phthalates, parabens, formaldehyde, and mercury that are utilized to produce many of the personal care products you obtain on store shelves. By themselves, each of these chemicals may present a risk to both human and environmental health.

But FDA officials and health experts all over the world are even more worried about the "cocktail effect" that may occur when these chemicals and toxins are mixed in the body and then subsequently in the environment. Daily exposure to these chemicals, combined with the various other substances found in your environment, may cause irreparable harm to both you and your baby.

Know Your Green Beauty Labels

So how can you make sure that the beauty products you use are healthy for you, your growing baby, and the environment? Read the labels. Sophie Uliano, an author of Gorgeously Green, estimates that women spend an average of 400 hours per year on their beauty routine. Indeed, it is worth spending five extra minutes at the store to ensure the products you choose are healthy for you and the environment.

You don't have to be a scientist to know which ingredients to look for and avoid your care products. It is simple — if you can pronounce the component and you wouldn't be afraid to eat it, it is more than likely safe to use on your skin. By contrast, if it sounds like a toxic chemical, then it probably is. Put that product down and move on to another.

Many companies have introduced nanoparticle-sized ingredients to their formulations. Nanoparticles allow ingredients to permeate the skin more easily, boosting the product's effect. They are commonly used in sunscreens and lotions to improve absorption. But since of their small size, they may become uncontrollable and unpredictable in the body. Make sure your skincare products are labeled nano-free.

Ingredients to Look For

Want to make sure your care products are safe? Look for ingredients, such as these, that you can read and that you wouldn't be afraid to eat (not that your shampoo will be delicious):

- Aloe Vera
- Beeswax
- Cocoa butter
- Essential oils
- Glycerin
- Herbs (green tea, chamomile, and lavender)

- Honey
- Lanolin
- Lemon
- Plant-based oils (almond, apricot, coconut, grape seed, jojoba bean, macadamia nut, olive, sesame, and tea tree)
- Vitamins
- Witch hazel

These ingredients are not only safe and healthy for you to use; they are also likely to be as or more effective than their synthetic chemical counterparts.

Ingredients to Avoid

Most commercial beauty products contain a few harsh and toxic ingredients that are anything but beautiful. Take five seconds to understand the label and put down any product that includes the following ingredients:

- BHA
- Formaldehyde
- Fragrance
- Lead
- Mercury
- Parabens
- Petroleum distillates
- Phthalates
- Polyethylene glycol

- Sodium Laurel Sulfate
- Toluene

These chemicals are deemed the most detrimental to human and environmental health. Here's why.

BHA. BHA, or beta hydroxy acid, is a preservative used in some skincare products. It is intended to reduce fine lines and wrinkles and other effects of aging. It may be listed as BHA, salicylic acid, salicylate, or sodium salicylate. It is also known as willow extract or beta-hydroxy butanoic acid. Others may even know it as tropic acid, or trethocanic acid. According to the Environmental Working Group (www.ewg.org), BHA has linked to certain types of cancer and organ system toxicity.

Formaldehyde. Also known as formalin, DMDM hydantoin, diazolidine urea, and quaternium-15, formaldehyde is found in eye shadows, mascaras, and other cosmetics. According to the National Toxicology Program, formaldehyde is a likely human carcinogen. Formaldehyde can be immersed through the skin and nails.

Products labeled "unscented" are not necessarily free from chemical fragrances. Often, these products just use more synthetic chemicals to mask their original odor. Look for products labeled fragrance-free and carefully check the ingredient list to ensure no fragrances are included in the formula.

Mercury. Your health care provider may have talked to you about the importance of limiting the amount of seafood you eat while pregnant to minimize your exposure to mercury. But he may not have mentioned that it is also possible to be exposed to mercury in your personal care products. Also known as thimerosal, mercury is found in individual eye drops and some makeup products, such as mascara and eye shadow.

Just since a product is labeled natural or all-natural does not mean that it is. Many beauty products that claim to contain botanic ingredients only have a small number of natural ingredients combined with chemicals. Skincare products only need to include 1 percent natural ingredients to be called realistic.

Petroleum distillates. Petroleum and petroleum derivates are commonly found in cold creams, lipsticks, lip protection, baby creams, and eye shadows. Petrolatum distillates can cause allergic reactions in sensitive individuals. And their production leads to the depletion of petroleum, a nonrenewable resource, and contributes to global warming.

Phthalates. Phthalates are synthetic, human-made substances used in the cosmetics industry to stabilize fragrances and make their aromas last longer. These chemicals have also been related to some frightening health risks, such as hormone disruption and reproductive changes known to cause congenital disabilities, sperm damage, infertility, and the feminization of baby boys. Dibutyl and trimethylphenyl phthalates have been banned in the European Union but not in the United States.

Polyethylene glycol. Polyethylene glycol, also known as propylene glycol, isopropyl alcohol, and butylene glycol, is used in cleansers and as a thickening agent in several skincare products. It is an acidic ingredient used to dissolve grease. It is the same ingredient used in oven cleaner.

Sodium lauryl sulfate. It has also been identified as sodium dodecyl sulfate or SDS, sodium laurel sulfate. It is a foaming agent that may be hazardous and is often contaminated with the known carcinogenic 1,4 dioxane. It is commonly found in sudsy beauty products like shampoo, bubble bath, soap, and toothpaste.

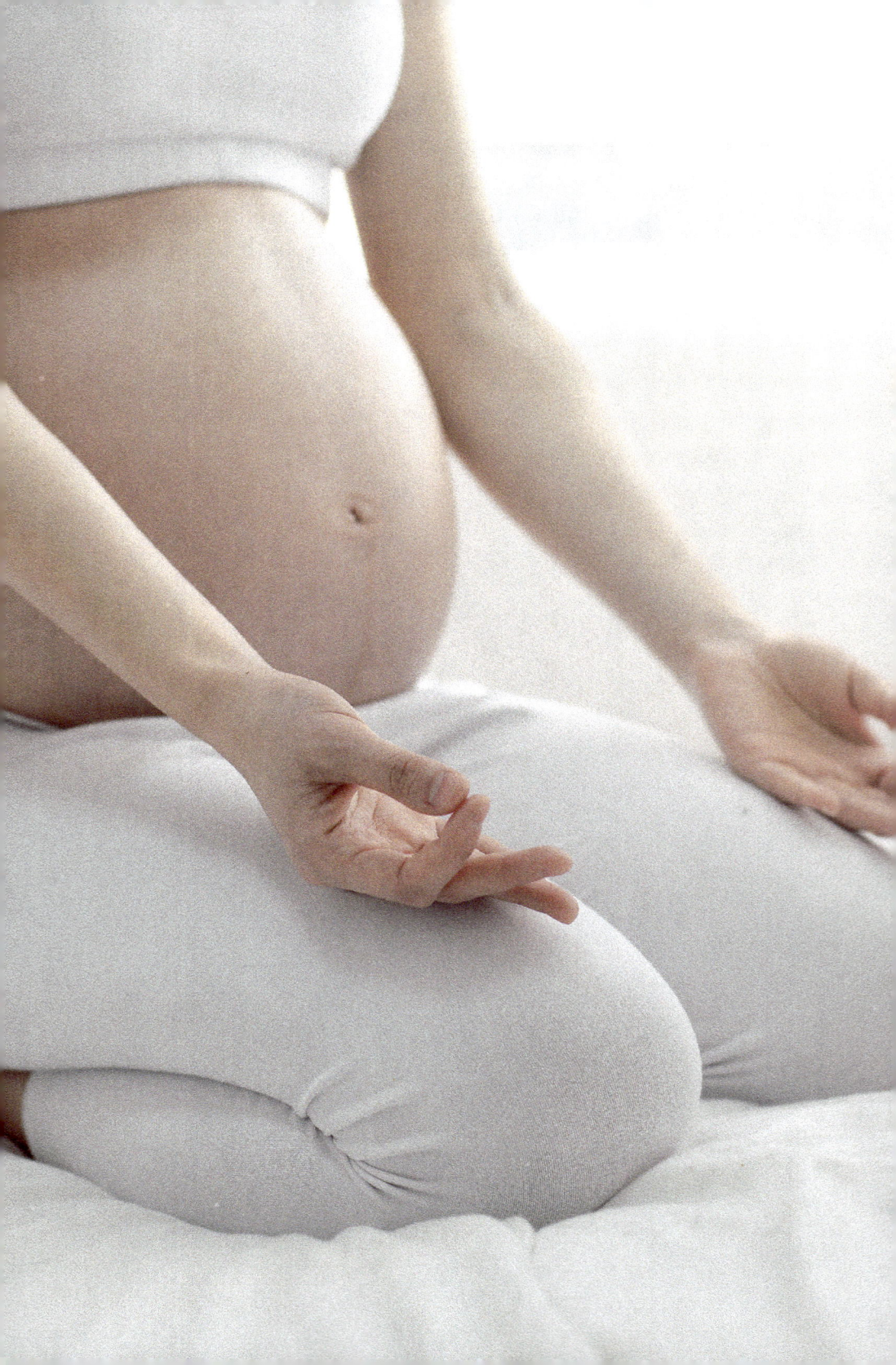

Chapter 17: Yoga and Childbirth

Yoga is a technique that can enhance skills for the preparation of labor. It helps to encourage the development of skills useful in parenting and any personal, physical, and emotional aspects of life. It helps activate the parasympathetic nervous system by stimulating the relaxation response discussed later in this book. Yoga connects the mind and body through postures, breath, and mindful awareness. It truly exercises the body, mind, and spirit, making it highly recommended during pregnancy. Learning how to control the breath and thoughts while holding unusual positions is excellent training for the physical event that is labor.

Yoga is for anyone and everyone and can be done in the comfort of home or at a studio or exercise facility. If you are new to the practice, be sure to listen to your body and not continue with a posture that causes pain. Pain and tension are two different things. When the muscles are tight, specific postures may seem uncomfortable; this is when the breath comes into play. Using the breath to go within and release the tension on each exhale allows your body to open up and experience the physical benefits that yoga has to offer. Prenatal yoga is designed to use the breath to help the expecting mother to focus on becoming aware of the sensations within the body.

Breathing Exercises

Breath is something perceived as so mundane, so voluntary, that it is often taken for granted. Breathing techniques are essential to practice during pregnancy to become familiar with conscious breathing when it is time for labor. Through moments of stress, our breathing typically becomes rapid and shallow, resulting in less oxygen circulating through the body and tense muscles. In the struggle, breathing techniques relaxed the mind, bring fresh oxygenated blood to the body/baby, and provide energy. Using the time to exercise the mind and body to breathe more efficiently helps all aspects of life and improves overall health and well-being.

-Deep Yogic Breathing is profound, even breaths through the nose and even deep exhalations through the nose. Practicing deep breathing requires complete growth and tightening of your lungs. This breath is used to refill healing qualities that are necessary to maintain harmony and balance. Being determined to fill and empty the lungs while also considering your facial muscles, making sure the muscles around the eyes and the jaw are relaxed. We carry stress in our face, hips, and shoulders, so intentionally relaxing one area tends to spread relaxation to those regions as well. This type of breathing exercise should be practiced daily in preparation for the big day and becomes useful to calm the mind in labor during contractions as the work progresses.

-Cleansing Breath follows the same head as deep yogic breathing but has a substantial emphasis on the exhalation throughout the mouth instead of the nose. This breath is used to clear gone tension, irritation, and negative thoughts and emotions. Take your interest in those tense or negative feelings and imagine they are being blown away with each breath as you exhale forcefully through the mouth. Cleansing Breath helps to clear carbon dioxide from your lungs and encourages the body to relax. This type of breathing exercise should not be practiced for long periods, but it can be practiced for 4-5 breaths to release negative emotions or tension. It becomes useful to regroup and release in between contractions.

Tips When Beginning Yoga

1. Listen to your body and modify postures as needed. Don't go past your limits; yoga is about body awareness; not about how flexible you are. Be accepting of the fact that where you are today is exactly where you are supposed to be. Every day will be different, but the important thing is that you try for this mind, body, and breath union, not how perfectly or profoundly you hold the asanas.

2. Remember to breathe. I know it sounds funny, but when we are in unusual, uncomfortable positions, it is common to compromise the breath. Even inhalations and exhalations through the nose help to keep your body and mind steady and calm. It also helps to be conscious of your facial muscles. If the jaw is clenched and the eyes are scrunched, it is common for the breath to be shallow and restricted. Relaxing the face helps to normalize breathing patterns.

3. Just do it! Like I mentioned before, it's not about how great you are at yoga; what matters is that you try to practice. Just like everything else, the more you practice, the better you become. Yoga is a great way to nourish, stretch, and lubricate your body, giving it an internal massage. Connecting with the mind, body, and breath regularly is vital for health and wellbeing. Another

great thing is that even if you don't have much time, a simple yoga stretch can have great rewards.

Chapter 18: Visualization and Childbirth

Visualizing your ideal birth experience is another necessary precursor to achieving it. Have you heard about mirror neurons? They're the nerve cells in your brain that begin to fire regardless of whether you do an activity, watch someone make a move, or merely visualize doing that activity yourself. It only begins to illustrate the power of the mind/body connection and how much your thoughts can affect your physiology.

Capitalizing on this, we have a concrete way to practice labor contractions (sometimes called surges) during pregnancy, even before experiencing them in labor and birth: spend time simply visualizing your ideal natural birth experience. How do you see yourself breathing, relaxing, chanting, singing, moaning, dancing, moving, etc., in your mind's eye? Can you visualize where you are, who is around you, and how you might like to respond to the sensations that come?

Ideally, you will want to dedicate time each day to thoughtfully visualizing your ideal natural birth experience. You'll imagine the specifics of how you'll give birth. Simply visualizing the birth, exactly how you would like it to happen, is extremely powerful. Even though every last detail of what you envision is unlikely to come to fruition, the act of anticipating these details will help you set the intention of how your birth will play out. You may do this exercise in any way that feels helpful for you.

For example, when I visualized my intended home birth, I only pictured myself in my home. I knew there was constantly the possibility that I'd have to transfer to the hospital, and I was OK with that, but I didn't want to spend time visualizing what a birth at the hospital might look like. I simply focused on images of myself laboring, moaning, vocalizing at home, in my bed, in my shower, in the birthing tub, in my clothes, my sheets, my food, etc. In short, I pictured myself in my familiar surroundings.

If you plan your natural birth in a hospital or birthing center, you might consider taking a tour of the space. Many hospitals will let you schedule a time to see their labor and delivery rooms, get a sense of how to get into the building/navigate the hallways and elevators, etc., and casually even meet a few providers.

It can do wonders for helping you envision your birthing environment. If you cannot take a tour, visualize as many details about yourself as you can.

For example:

- Where in your house (or outside your home) will you spend early labor before you go to the hospital or birthing center?
- If labor is progressing slowly, might you take a walk around the neighborhood?
- Where will you feel the least disturbed so that you can focus during early labor?
- What are you wearing when you visualize your labor and birth? A hospital gown. Your clothes? Your birthday suits?
- Who is with you? You can't always control who is on shift once at the hospital, but you can control which family members and hired birth attendants are by your side.

- Are the members of the birth team talking with you between contractions, or do you think you'll prefer to stay quiet?
- How are you breathing?
- Are you moaning or vocalizing, or are you not making much noise?
- Are you listening to music, guided mediation or visualization apps, or guided birth breathing? Are you utilizing earphones or a speaker system?

You can also spend a little time visualizing how you'll handle possible complications. How might you communicate with your team if something changes and your labor doesn't go according to plan? How can you continue to feel autonomous if you need to have an intervention? Hint: Stay informed about what is going on, weigh the risks, and seek the advice of your chosen birth team members. After all, you chose them because you trust them wholeheartedly. If you make decisions mindfully every step of the way, you will feel in charge of the progression of your baby's birth, even if there are lucky stumbling blocks. Visualize how you might handle challenging situations so that it is still within the realm of your ideal. But a phrase of warning: do not get wrapped up in visualizing possible complications.

Set aside time each day (five to twenty minutes) just for visualizing your ideal birth.

The first time, mostly, if done during early pregnancy, may take longer for images to pop up. Close your eyes for a minute and guess what ideas arise when you think about birth. Let any images that emerge speak to you. Even if you visualize birthing somewhere completely impractical—some sort of mystical or spiritual place—if it feels good, then it's the right image to hold onto. You can return to these places, these visualizations in your mind, to bring yourself a sense of calm. Once you find some mental pictures that feel good, keep returning to these images to solidify them in your psyche.

After you've done a few visualization sessions, some of the images will begin to stick with you more than others. Use the following questions to help embed the most powerful images firmly in your imagination. Write out the answers to help make the images even more powerful.

- Where are you birthing in your mind's eye?
- Who is around you during your early labor, transition, and pushing stages?
- What different body positions are you in during labor?
- What are you wearing?
- Do you have music playing?
- What is the lighting in the room?
- What time of day feels ideal for you?
- How warm or cold is it?

When you repeat your visualizations, allow for new positive birth images and ideas to emerge. Once you have a stable view of how you envision the birth, spend your visualization time focusing on images reinforcing this vision. If you found any beautiful mental images that do not specifically pertain to your birth but bring you tranquility (e.g., being in a field of poppies with doves and unicorns), use these images as relaxation tools. When I did visualization exercises in preparation for my birth, I saw myself in a hot tub, sipping a glass of wine with a beautiful stone fireplace flickering gently in front of me. This image was so relaxing that it brought me immense pleasure to practice before my birth, and it became a safe space for me to go to in my mind during labor.

Preparation will undoubtedly help with your mental stamina during labor and, given the interplay between your mind and your body, it will likely benefit your physical energy as well.

Whether you're preparing to birth at home or a hospital or birthing center, use these visualizations to watch yourself in your ideal labor virtually. Can you start to see how strong and warrior-like you look? It is fantastic to work with you are doing! Commend your visualization-self for such strength, commitment, and passion.

In addition to committing to your natural childbirth, you will want to be intentional about how you speak about the coming labor. Words shape experience, so if you continually think and talk about pain, for example, you prime yourself to experience labor as painful.

In current years, as we have started to learn more about the power words have on our minds and bodies, there has been a shift toward using some new birth terms. For example, instead of "contractions," which implies tightness and restriction when you want to encourage relaxing and softening, the term "surges" is sometimes used. (This term was initially coined by the HypnoBirthing© method. It has been embraced by many in the natural birthing community.) Some women say they experience "sensations" instead of "pain." To be sure, many women describe these sensations as painful, but others don't.

You can think of your midwife or doctor as "attending the birth" and "catching" instead of "delivering" your baby. You and the baby are the ones birthing. Others are merely catching the baby as s/he arrives.

Similarly, let's avoid saying or thinking that your medical attendants know what to do to help or save you. You want to talk about yourself and other birthing women as being healthy and supremely capable. You are the expert of your own body; you should reinforce the belief that you and your body know what to do. (Even when this means handing yourself over to others.)

Even if you adopt this more positive language, I bet you'll still find yourself discussing uterine "contractions" or "pain" at one point or another—these terms are ingrained in our terminology and have infiltrated how we think about birth. And frankly, many people do experience the birthing process as painful, me included. But if you envision and describe yourself as having "surges" or "sensations" or "pressure" instead of pain during labor, it will go a long way toward changing your perspective and creating a positive frame of mind. Try it out. See how you feel using these words when you talk about the upcoming birth. Ultimately, you should always speak in a way that feels authentic to you.

When I experienced the peak of my surges during my daughter's birth, I once moaned, "This is hhhhoooorrriiiibbbbllleeee," only to find that my sensations became exponentially more painful as I uttered these words. Seriously. It was fiercely powerful to recognize just how much influence the mind has over the body. As I recovered from that surge, I tried to correct myself by whimpering, "I mean, that was awesome," much to the amusement of my husband and doula. I then worked to keep my mind positive and ride the surges without focusing so intensely on the sensations. I did not make the same mistake again.

Remember, also that you should try to avoid people who use negative language. Especially when talking about having a natural birth—which I encourage you to speak of proudly! —you might find that people will give you unwanted opinions or want to tell you scary birth stories. I'm not sure what causes us to do this to one another. Assuming they mean no harm, I suspect it's intended as a heartfelt reminder that birth is a massive event that is hard to anticipate and unlike any other. For many people, the unknown is scary, and they may feel they are supportive by trying to give you a heads-up about its difficulty and overwhelming essence. But each of us is unique; our experiences are unique; our bodies are individual; our babies are unique, and our births are uncommon. Don't be afraid to speak in words that taste best on your tongue and fall best on your ears. You are in charge.

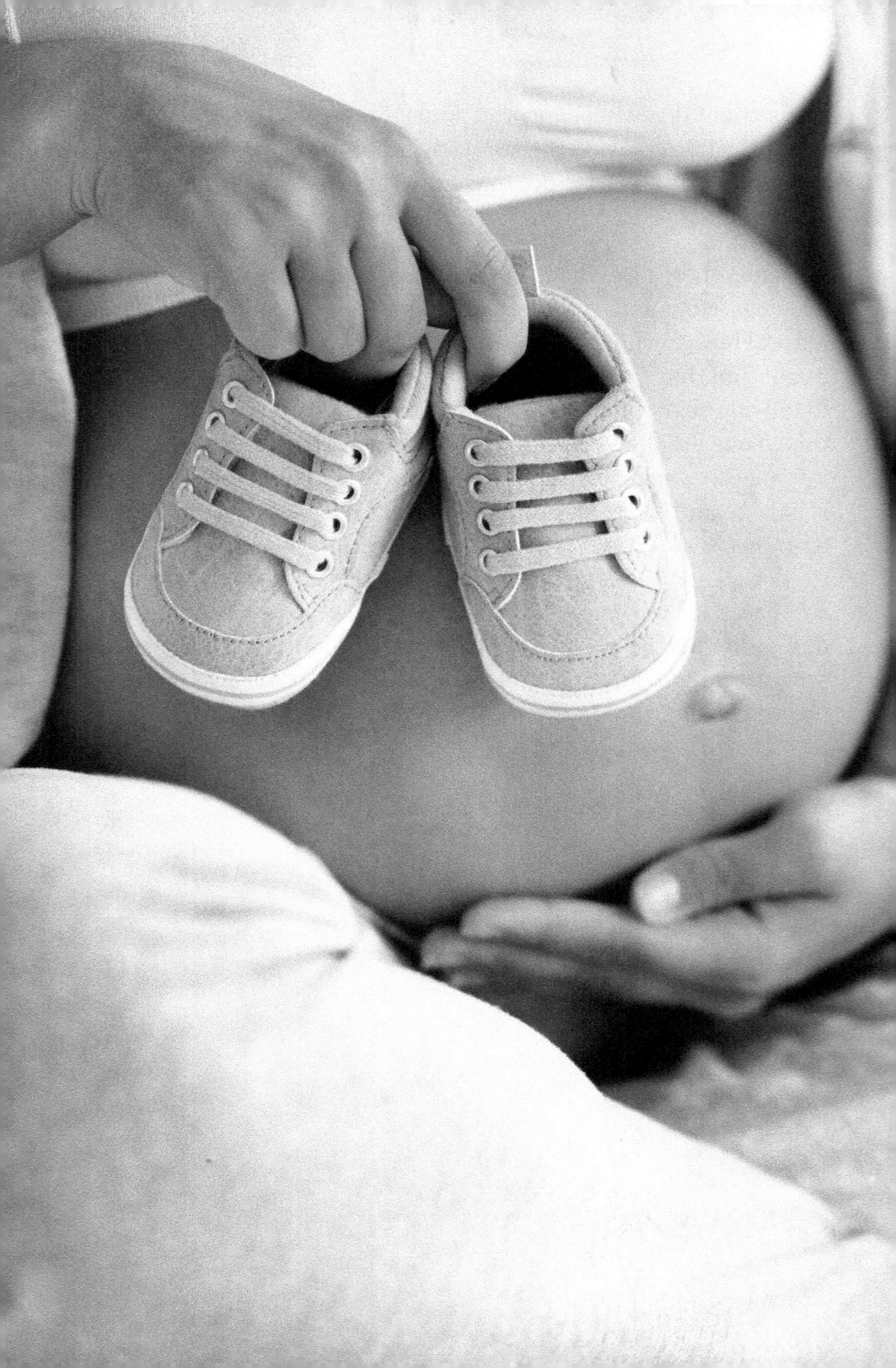

Chapter 19: In Control

I had an epiphany the initial moment I heard Dr Phil say, "If you buy the ticket, you take the ride."

Over the years, I've seen numerous parents try toward better birth with a strong desire and heartfelt changes, only to have it come apart at the seams. Why? Two reasons, mainly.

They are making decisions they know with their heads are right, but their hearts are afraid to believe more is possible. Beliefs, unconscious fears, and faulty assumptions lay in wait for a moment to spring up. Modern obstetric care seems to justify everything, which gives ample opportunity for doubt to creep in.

A mother is encouraged to have an ultrasound at eight weeks. She's hesitant, having heard there could be risks to early ultrasound, including increased miscarriage, but her nurse-midwife tells her that they have to determine a due date. Not knowing that a.) due date is irrelevant at this point b.) a due date should be a 'due month' and c.) this will do nothing to change her care, she agrees.

She is told there is 'something possibly wrong with the yolk sac,' and she will need another ultrasound at 12 weeks. If there is 'something wrong with the yolk sac,' she will probably miscarry. If she doesn't, a resulting anomaly could be severe enough. She might be counseled to abort. If she chooses not to, nothing can be done to rectify the situation. So, either way, her care doesn't change.

It sounds as if there is medical justification, but there is none other than the concern her care provider has regarding liability. There are specific procedures and protocols (in fact, most of those regarding hospital birth) that have nothing—not one thing—to do with actual safety and everything to do with the advice of a lawyer.

Consider a woman having had a previous cesarean for a failed induction. Her doctor insists that 'for her safety,' they will have to induce this time if she goes past her due date. If it looks like the baby will be significant (via ultrasound, of course, which can be two pounds off in either direction!) or if she doesn't deliver during daylight hours.

Even though none of these recommendations are evidence-based, the induction is refuted by the very study often cited as the reason for the guidance. (Mona Lydon-Rochelle et al., 2001) This study says not that VBAC is unsafe, but that chemically induced or augmented VBAC is unsafe. But the mother, in our example, is convinced that she should concede. After all, it sounds like there is a medical indication. It is a case of CYA on the part of the hospital, not mom's concern.

A birth story passed my desk of a woman who was induced because her doctor thought she 'looked ready,' and by ultrasound, her baby looked to be about 8 ½ pounds, which he deemed to be getting 'too big.'

After sufficiently frightening her with dire predictions of a stuck baby, she consented to an induction. The parents felt the doctor was terrific throughout the pregnancy and didn't feel they were pushed into an installation. As far as the parents were anxious, the doctor was just doing his job and looking out for their best interest. Never mind that induction is notorious for ending in unnecessary cesareans (Wilson, Effken, & Butler, 2012; Ehrenthal, Xiaozhang & Strobino, 2010) without improving outcomes, or that ultrasound is notorious for being highly undependable at weight estimation.

Her baby is born after difficult labor (again, a known consequence of induction) weighing in at only 6 pounds 10 oz., under 19 inches long, with an estimated gestational age of 35 or 36 weeks. This prematurity was not only preventable but created by the provider. The parents will be lucky if there are no developmental delays for their child, which is why we purport to try to prevent premature births.

Another case of preventable prematurity touched on earlier was the woman with twins. Her doctor had warned her throughout her whole pregnancy that she should expect to deliver early. By the time she was 30 weeks along, she was told she 'might not make it to next week.'

Always the parents are making decisions based on one source of information that is hardly unbiased. It sounds as if there's medical justification, but is there? In pregnancy, more than anywhere else, it's essential to seek out other sources of information and second opinions. Yet, it is precisely here that such investigation into your health and well-being is most discouraged. Why?

Chapters leading up to this point have laid out a plan for avoiding the pitfalls the above parents encountered, so you are one step ahead in this area. But what of those parents at the beginning of the chapter who tried so hard and were still sabotaged? What is the other reason the best of plans was ruined?

They were trying to fit a square peg into a round hole. This behavior comes from an underlying fear, the 'just in case' mentality. Still, it's the act of trying to make the medical model fit the midwifery model—or maybe even thinking that it's possible—that creates problems.

It sounds something like this: 'I know birth is a healthy, natural process, but [now ignore that and listen to what I believe] we want to have our first baby with Dr. So-and-so, just in case something happens." Thus, ensuring 'something' will happen only by the law of probability.

It usually plays out something like this:

Mr. & Mrs. Anybody is enlightened and intelligent expectant parents. They have read a dozen books and are in an independent childbirth class. They learn about informed consumerism, evidence-based care, and the consequences of inappropriate birth technology. They make a birth plan. They outline all of the things that are important to them. They take it to their doctor, who barely glances at it and says, "Yeah, sure, whatever you want…as long as there are no problems." Sounds reasonable so far, right?

Mr. & Mrs. Anybody know that midwives encourage ambulation (walking in labor), so they ask if that would be allowed for them. "Sure, we want to have you up and about… except for when we need to have you on the monitor, or of course, after you've had your pain relief."

"We won't be using pharmaceuticals." Mr. & Mrs. Anybody reminds him.

"Huh?" He looks up from their chart. "Oh, right. Ok, if you say so." He says with a grin.

Midwives provide perineal support. Will he? "Of course," he says, "unless I see that you need an episiotomy, at which time I assume you want me to do one instead of letting you rip wide open."

"Certainly!" Mrs. Anyone agrees. He must make that determination. After all, that's why they hired him.

"We'd like the cord to stop pulsing before being cut." the parents' request.

"Sure," The doctor amiably replies, "not a problem! Unless, of course, the baby needs to be resuscitated or you are hemorrhaging or something." He says in an off-hand manner as if it happens all the time.

"Of course." The parents say weakly, growing pale in the face as they picture these complications that must be so common that the doctor would mention them.

If 90% of communication is between the lines, these parents should be running, not walking, to the nearest exit. Instead, they tell themselves what a good thing is that they chose this doctor who will "let" them do what they want in labor. They have the 'best of both worlds' as far as they are concerned. They push down the feelings of unease that struggle to be acknowledged.

He tells them he is scheduling a triple test for next week, a gestational diabetes test for the week after, and an ultrasound for the week after that.

"We'd like to avoid further routine prenatal testing." The

parents again must remind him.

"Of course, you do!" he agrees. "I wouldn't suggest these if I didn't think they were important. You see, I'm concerned about your fundal height. The baby might not be growing as well as I'd like. So, we need to have that ultrasound." (He doesn't add that repeated ultrasound is implicated in intra-uterine growth retardation—the condition he supposedly is looking for) (Wagner, 1999.)

He continues, "The triple test is probably not necessary, but it's just a simple blood draw, no problem at all really. Not invasive. No reason not to do it if we can save you heartache down the road." (There is no mention of the fact this test has a high rate of false positives that could result in immeasurable heartache) (Graves, Miller, & Sellers, 2002)

Adding, "Gestational diabetes is treatable. If you have it, wouldn't you want to know so that you could prevent the high rate of stillbirth that occurs with diabetic mothers?" (Again, no explanation that the high rate of stillbirth is with women who have a preexisting condition or history of diabetes in the family, who may be exhibiting signs or symptoms of manifesting the condition. Also, no mention that the American Diabetes Association advises against routine testing of healthy women because there is no improvement in outcomes). * If you were my wife, I'd want you to have it."

He's been so cooperative. They go along with it. One test leads to another. He may even agree that some of the tests aren't necessary unless. Somehow, there is always a reason that seems legitimate to have them done. Each ten-minute visit with Dr. Soand-so seems to build a relationship based on trust and full disclosure, yet they haven't given true informed on anything. They may get their dream birth, but I wouldn't bet on it. Even if a couple has avoided the vast majority of unnecessary technology through pregnancy, the caregiver who misuses or overuses technology will find a way to justify his presence at the birth somehow by the time all is said and done.

You buy the ticket; you take the ride. As Nancy Wainer says, "If you don't want surgery, don't go to a surgeon." It's not fair to the surgeon to expect him to practice midwifery. He's not a midwife. He's not trained in normalcy, and he's not geared to sit around doing anything until he's needed. The medical establishment is based on pathology. He's trained to do something anything! Going to a hospital and hiring a doctor, but telling them, "I'd like it to be as close to home birth as possible" (something they hear all the time) is an unrealistic expectation.

Remember, some doctors practicing in hospitals don't believe home birth is safe, despite all the contrary evidence. If they did, they'd be doing them. You aren't going to change their belief system in the short period of your pregnancy, so why would their behavior change? You have not altered their underlying assumptions about the very nature of birth, and you won't because all around them, they see 'evidence' to support their belief. Birth is a horrifying event in the hospital. When I have done a string of hospital labor support jobs without home births to balance them out, I've started to doubt the safety of birth. I can't blame them if that's all they see. I agree, Yikes!

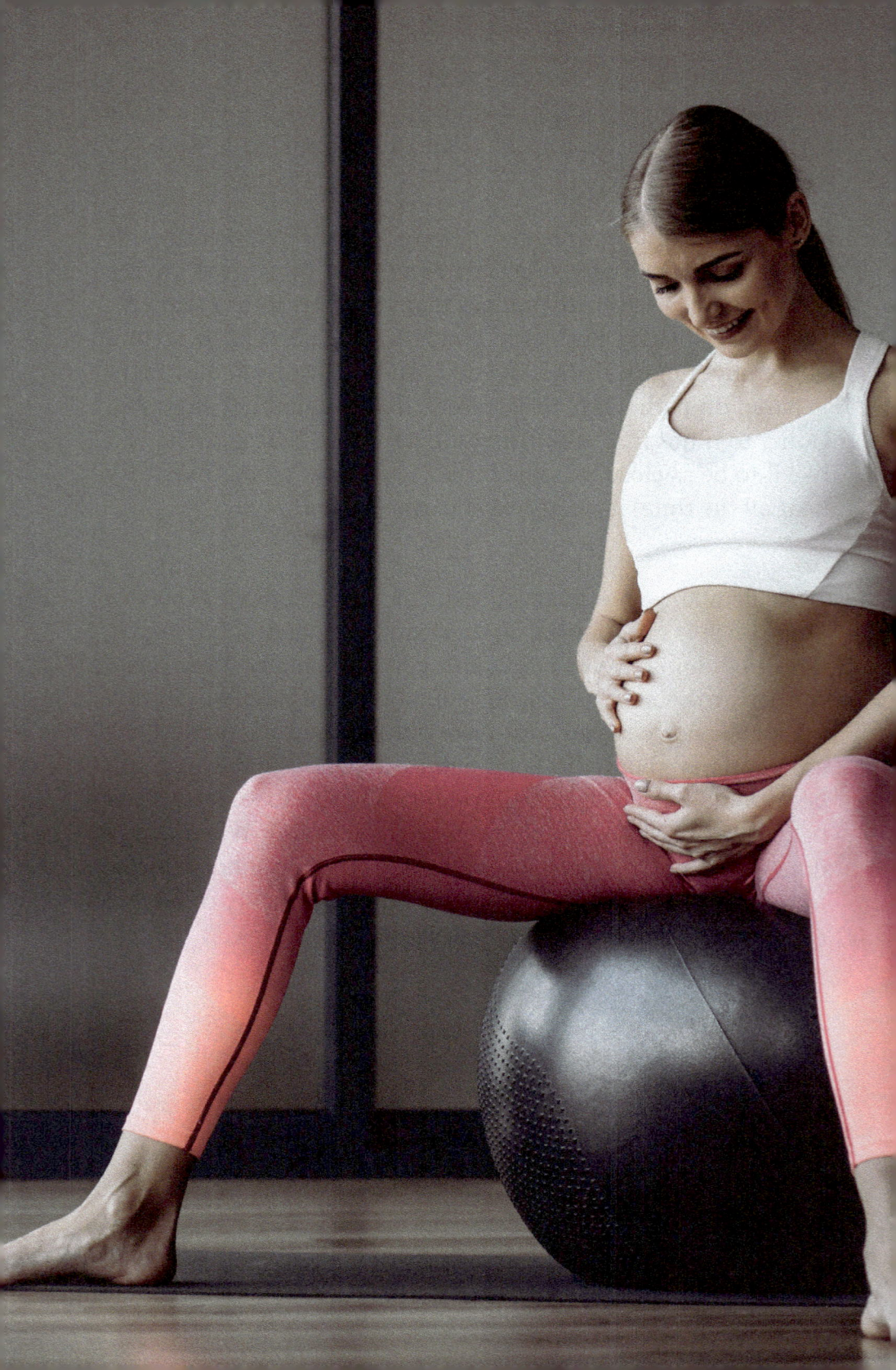

Chapter 20: Relaxation During Childbirth

The Importance of Relaxation at the Birth

After learning how to get rid of the fear of birthing, you must learn how to relax deeply and quickly. Later, in this book, I will teach you several methods that you can use to achieve this, but why is this so important? For starters, it's a lot easier for your body to bring you your baby when your body is relaxed; all the doctors, nurses, and midwives that I've consulted in my years of doing this have all agreed. However, learning how to relax is not enough. What is ultimately more important than just relaxation is learning how to relax quickly and powerfully on command.

At the beginning of the birthing process, the contractions will be further apart than when the birth progresses. As you get closer to delivering your baby, the contractions will be 1-2 minutes apart. You don't have the comfort of taking 20, 15, or even 10 minutes to relax because as you try to relax, the contraction may throw you off balance, so even 10 minutes is too long. Therefore, quick relaxation is essential. You need to get into a quick, deep state of relaxation before the intensity of the contraction builds. It implies that you ought to get into a state of relaxation as quickly as 1 minute, which is possible when you work with the subconscious mind.

Throughout the pages of this book, I can teach you several

techniques that can help you relax on command. Still, unfortunately, I can't work with your subconscious mind as I do in the course or CD's, so you have to focus on practicing how to relax quickly on your own, and as often as you can, unless you decide to take the course.

The Contradiction

The exceptionally first thing that you must learn about mental relaxation is that you can't actively relax your mind. Of course, this sounds like a contradiction, I just got through telling you that working with the mind instead of the body in relaxation is most important, and now I'm telling you that you can't relax it, to begin with. Why?

You can't relax your mind; you must allow it to relax. In other words, you can't actively relax your mind, but you can passively relax it, and this is what we usually do when we get deep relaxation or when we go to sleep. While you go to bed in the evening, you don't try to go to sleep. You just fall asleep. You know, at some point, if you "try" to fall asleep, you just end up staying awake, don't you and boy do it get frustrating.

The way you fall asleep is by focusing on relaxation, your body, perhaps the things you did during the day, and letting the thoughts drop off one at a time. It usually happens naturally, and when a few thoughts drop away, then more, and more, and more, and before you know it, you are waking up.

In this process of falling asleep, you don't usually actively relax your mind because if you force your mind to relax, it generates more thoughts. Suppressing thoughts only causes the mind to panic and bring up more thoughts. It is because relaxation is a passive process, and thinking is an active one. Make sense?

Do this for fun; try to stop thinking and see how long it takes before you begin to think again. Go ahead, do it now. You probably didn't get past a few seconds, right? When you thought about whether you were thinking or not, you started to think again. It is because relaxation is a passive process, and thinking is an active one. If you try to relax, you are active, meaning that you are not relaxing. Try this instead. Ask yourself, "what is my next thought?" What happens? Many people experience their mind freezing for a few moments. The reasons are more profound than what we can get into this work. For now, it's just a fun exercise.

The Job of the Mind

The mind's job is to think and thinking convinces us that we exist. If we are not thinking and solving something like a problem, whether good or bad, we have the illusion that we've ceased to exist. You may say, "That's not true." I shout, "Don't take my phrase for it. Give it some thought."

What would you do with yourself if you weren't solving your or someone else's problem? What if I could wave a magic wand and make all your problems go away where you wouldn't have to deal with even one? In the beginning, many people say, "that's great," but then many think about that question and say, "If I didn't have a problem, my life would be so boring."

Do you get my point? The mind likes to think, and stopping mental activity is not part of our list. Besides, today's woman is so active and so productive that stopping the mind for a while may not feel productive, so the best thing you can do for your mind when relaxing is to take a completely passive approach.

I feel I must address that some people always like to control and worry over the thought of being so passive. If you resemble this in any way, then I will remind you that controlling everything is impossible, and if the mind can't relax, isn't this already a loss of control? You may think of mental passivity as taking a passive role in being able to gain control. In other words, you are letting go of a desire to control, to gain control.

It's letting go of the illusion that being in control of everything is possible (in other words, you can't be in control of everything) and allow for more control in your life by creating that balance of being active and passive. The active is living your everyday life in a typical active fashion. The passive is giving yourself that much needed time to relax to recuperate and restore your balance, actually becoming passive is part of the balance that we need in our lives.

How to Reach a State of Mental Passivity

You already know that your mind will not clear, stop or relax for long upon request. It is possible but doing this requires much practice. However, you can clear your mind with minimal practice by winning the mind at its own game. What I entail by this is that the mind must stay occupied at all times, so you need to use that principle to take greater control of your mind and keep your mind busy with something pleasant. Using the senses (like hearing) works so well because you stimulate the brain, causing the mind to think or focus on what you are listening to.

Try this…take the index and middle finger of one of your hands and quickly begin to tap alternating the index and middle finger. As you tap, look, and your fingers, and notice that your mind becomes so busy focusing on the tapping that you are not thinking about anything else. Neat huh?

Why did your mind stop thinking about other things? The reason is that the mind can only concentrate on one thing at a time. Besides, you gave your mind a focus, and that helped it to only think about that one thing that you were doing, which helped the mind clear.

Another thing you can do is listen to something pleasant like the sound of waves on the beach live or from a CD. It doesn't have to be waves; it can be birds, the wind, rainstorms, or meditative music. It can also be a dull background sound like the hum of the air conditioner or a fan. Many of these pleasant sounds can be found on the Internet or apps for free.

Besides using the auditory senses, you can also utilize the visual senses to focus your eyes or sight on a pleasant scene. You can choose the picture of a beach, forest, or any lovely scenery. You can even focus on a spot on the wall or ceiling. It will cause your mind to focus intently on one thing and clear thoughts. I have nice pictures in my office so that my patients can focus on them before they go into that relaxed hypnotic state. The picture does not usually put someone into a trance. Instead, it helps a person focus his or her mind in preparation for trance.

The point here is to keep your mind occupied with something pleasant just as it always keeps itself occupied. This way, frightening thoughts don't enter the mind, and you are not giving up control; you are merely shifting your focus. Shifting focus is a lot more palatable for us because it incorporates something that we do all the time anyway.

Another way of calming the mind or making it more passive is by using feelings. You can use your mind to become aware of your hands or feet. Usually, the extremities are much easier felt. Do this exercise by paying particular attention to the hands or feet and feel for a subtle tingling sensation. If you sit still and bring your full attention to one of the extremities, you will feel it. Most people that I've worked with can do this successfully. Some are not able to at first, but then areas they open their awareness.

Doing this exercise is excellent and puts you in the present moment. In the Wizard of Oz, the character named Dorothy said, "There is no place like home," and to add to Dorothy's words, there is no moment like the present. In the present moment, there is nothing but peace because there's an intense fixation of NOW. Focusing on the present moment by becoming deeply aware of yourself is a great way to let go of extraneous annoying thoughts. It's a practice that is easy but may seem difficult to some because they are not doing anything. For those that need to be in control, it's an excellent means of letting go of some of that strong desire to be in control. Its' also another tool that you can use in relaxation.

I mention you to an excellent book on this subject titled The Power of Now by Eckhart Tolle. One time I did a weekend seminar with one of Tolle's students, and it was one of the most powerful weekends I've ever had. The emphasis of the workshop was to teach people how to put themselves in and stay in the moment. The exercises were straightforward yet extremely powerful.

It does require time and practice because the mind's focus tends to stray, but again it is achievable. All you need is persistence. It's vital to keep in mind that if the mind strays, gently bring it back to the center as the mind will fight you if you try to force it. As you are doing this, you may also focus on the rise and fall of the chest as air moves through the lungs; this is meditative.

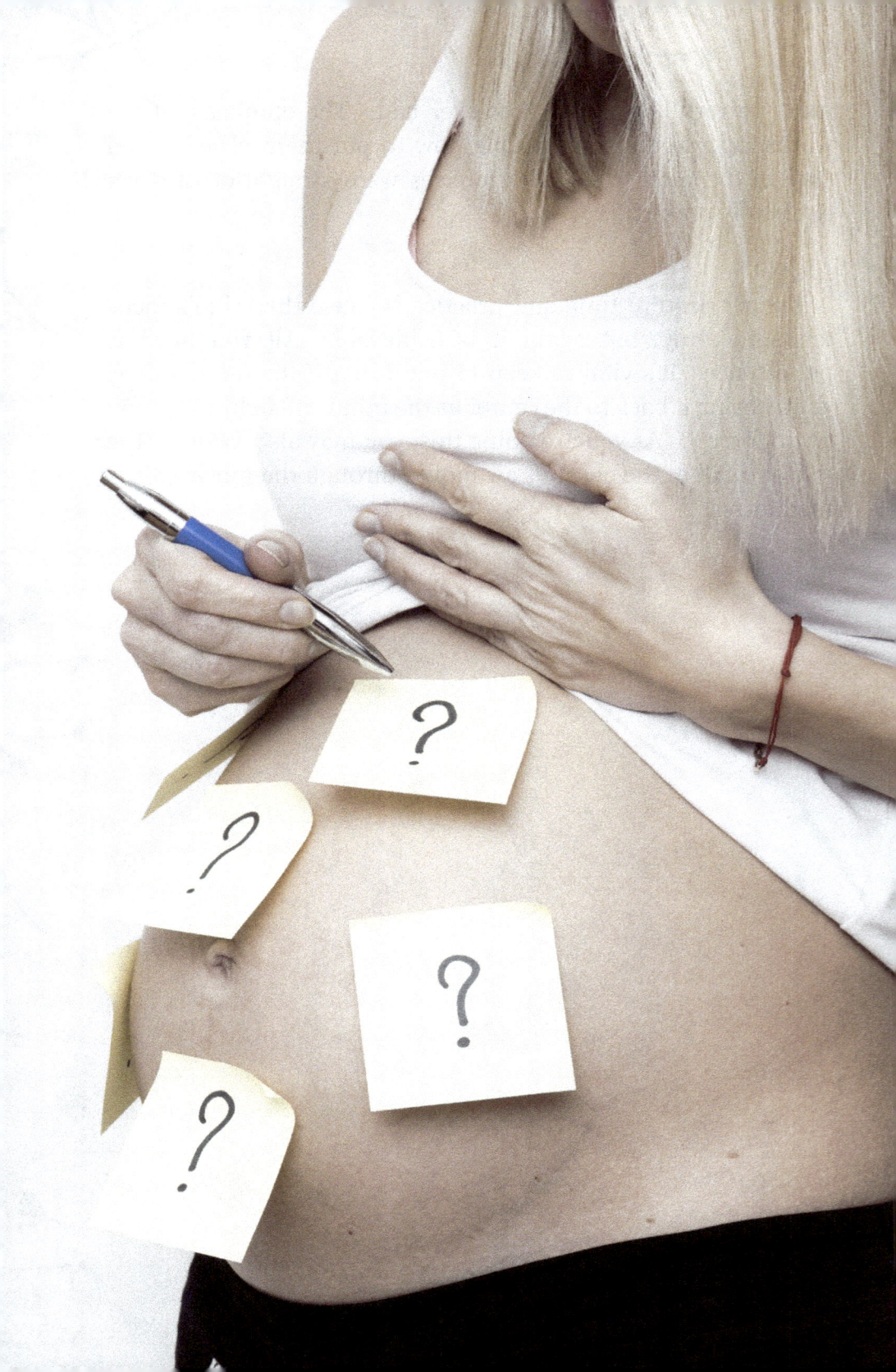

Chapter 21: Sources of Childbirth Pangs

Unnatural Human Foods

(Meat, starches, sugar, dairy, chemical additives, and preservatives)

Your body needs fluidity. Starchy, ~stiffy~ foods with cause a STIFF and painful body. Thus, the way to avoid and eliminate the chances of pain throughout pregnancy is to ensure your body's elasticity by being fluid (full of living waters); indeed, you will be forever glad you did! Unnatural human foods can also cause the following:

- Unnatural rapid growth (fetus/baby, and mother)
- Unnatural bone solidification; harden stored waste accumulation within organs and tissues.
- Emotional overeating, "Comfort Eating" (unconscious guilt eating)

Many of those preservatives, additives, and other food chemicals are found in almost ALL store-bought packaged food, EVEN vegan pre-packaged foods, and some supposedly raw packaged foods. More than likely, consuming these things can and will cause our bodies to become numb, stiff, hardened, or DEADENED.

- Can a deadened uterus contract on its own to release a baby with ease?
- Can a deadened, malfunctioning body produce a lively baby?

- Can a deadened body enjoy the pleasure of being in conception?

- Can a deadened body rid itself of the normal "so-called" maternal issues?

The answer is NO.

Restrictive Birthing Positions

Lying flat on your back with your knees cocked out is not the ideal birthing position. It's familiar but not the most comfortable. During birth, significantly, if not in a hospital, move until the baby is swirling down the birth canal. Moving during pregnancy helps to eliminate pain because your body is focused on moving and being non-restrictive.

The truth is when your body is fully ready for delivery, regardless of what birthing position you're in (although I recommend ones that allow for free movement); the baby will slither out without difficulty.

Fearful Thoughts and Environments

Nothing places pain in pregnancy like poisoned people, places, and things. What you decide to let in your inner and physical environment will either make you or break you. Remaining centered is one of the critical components that will assist with laboring painlessly. How can you maintain your peace if you're not at peace, firstly? Trying to have a painless pregnancy in and of itself is not the average pregnancy expectation of most mothers. So be discrete when relating this goal to others. Only share with those who want to support you because what you need now is only support and love. Fear is another factor that contributes to pain during delivery. Your body can't fully perform at an optimal level if it's not free from fear. Do all that you can to refrain from the cold, fear-laden tense environment, and people that stress and cause stiffness, not relaxing, comforting peace, and calm experiences to naturally open your womb with ease.

Fear and Womb Restriction

Dilation is needed for the baby to be born through the womb. The cervix must be able to stretch and open effectively. As labor nears, the cervix may begin to stretch and open to prepare for the passage of the baby through the womb. How fast this happens to vary from mother to mother (depending on personal lifestyle, nutrition, and choices). However, if fear is around, it can cause slow dilation and super slow labor and delivery. Your womb will naturally close to birthing related fear or fear in general. Some women's cervical dilation can indeed have reached 10 centimeters and brought down back to 5 centimeters due to fearful birthing thoughts and unpleasant birthing situations.

Forced Unnatural Pushing & Digging into the Womb Canal(s)

If you want pain during childbirth, push before your child is ready to be birthed. Your body needs no assistance with the opening. It does just fine on its own when left alone. Have you ever tried to have a bowel movement that wasn't ready to come out? I'm quite sure it wasn't very pleasurable. But instead of your "bottom" being sore, it will be your womb as a substitute.

It's never a good idea to force the course of a river or a baby in this instance. The same applies to eat nourishment. The fruit of a tree only tastes good once it's ripe. The unripe fruit is bitter, can damage the body, and doesn't taste great. Unripe babies are fragile and sickly. So, do you, child, a favor and wait it out.

Most unnatural pushing occurs in hospitals where your pregnancy is being dictated by "others." The baby will surely let you know when it's ready to arrive. We don't have to decide on it. The baby is well capable of doing it on its own. Let's not interfere and cause the body more pain. Plus, unnatural pushing is painful. Save yourself the pain and relax and be patient. Wait on the child! When the baby is eager to come out, it signals that the womb has reached its stretching point to allow the "little one" to slide on through. Birthing children is much easier when our womb has reached its stretching point. A lot of women are not able to reach this point due to premature pushing. And again, this method causes lots of pain.

Relationships

- Is it safe, secure, and bonded with trust and divine purpose? If no relationship with the father exists, does the mother have closure and a clear free mind regarding the matter, i.e., no guilt, regret, anger, etc. (understands that the child's coming has a purpose for life).

- Who is the mother's support system? How are those relationships?

A good support team is essential in the line of pregnancy duty. Having loving relationships where everyone understands and supports the decisions being made is essential. You can't have a painless pregnancy if entangled on an emotional rollercoaster and perceiving life to have dealt us a bad hand because of relationship status. God doesn't make womb "mistakes." The blessing in the depths of your womb is a gift. So, if your relationship status is rocky with the father of your child, make sure that it's not with your Maker. After all, the Creator just gave you a gift. The least you can say is thank-you! Having a strong foundational relationship with God will create more peace and less pain.

Intimacy, Pregnancy, and Miscarriages

A lot of times, this is a topic most women rather not discuss, especially while pregnant. The thought of not having sexual intercourse with their mate for nine months may not digest well to them. It brings up another vital point to consider, copulation during pregnancy, especially the latter stages. Copulation is another thing that can bring on the premature breaking of the water, among other issues. Full throttle copulation during the mid-latter stage's pregnancy can be hazardous for both mother and child. It has been a hidden, and often undocumented source (most health professionals have deemed it to be a "healthy act throughout pregnancy/conception") of many premature births, miscarriages, hysterectomies, and can have a significant impact on mental development and can contribute to developmental disorders/dysfunction.

Copulation is a spiritual and electrical force with rules and laws that are built into its function. For example, when a woman's stimulated through copulation, the womb electrifies and prepares to receive spiritual input for life. This stimulation also causes the uterus (inner womb) to receive and assimilate that input, but what about when there's already a child developing within the uterus. We must consider what happens when it's opened and if/how this may affect the womb and the developing child…? So, this, too, is something that you should pay close attention to or begin to observe more closely the responses of the inner womb and child to copulation, especially during the mid-latter stages of pregnancy.

Although many say that intercourse is safe during pregnancy, mothers should consider hoe safe. They knew that the womb contracts during orgasms signal a red light to consider opting out of or slowing down with intimate relations. It's a known fact that having intercourse later in pregnancy can bring on labor, and the same is actual at the beginning and the middle of pregnancy. The purpose of intercourse is procreation. And yes, our Maker has made it enjoyable, but once that seed has been planted, shouldn't we wait until harvest to gather the goods and plant another one in that same spot? After a woman conceives, shouldn't she stop trying to conceive until the baby is birthed? The sperm is a great penetrator. If a woman continually engages in intercourse, over a period, could the sperm damage the water bag and breach it causing premature births and miscarriages? These are all terrific questions to ask ourselves.

Although research is sparse concerning intercourse and miscarriages, women should listen to their bodies while pregnant and do as told.

Many women say that " My baby is far too low, and it feels like it is about to drop" far too soon in pregnancy. It can partially be due to consistent intercourse. If both partners are thrusting hard, the placenta can detach, releasing the baby soon after. When pregnant mothers are in rear-ended accidents, due to the force of the push from the opposing car from behind, the placenta can detach if the force of the hit was powerful. The same applies to intercourse in this matter. So, mothers, just being mindful of your actions because no one will advocate discontinuing sexual activity while pregnant. But if it begins to feel uncomfortable, your womb begins to feel weak or the baby balls up tightly while engaging and afterward, STOP.

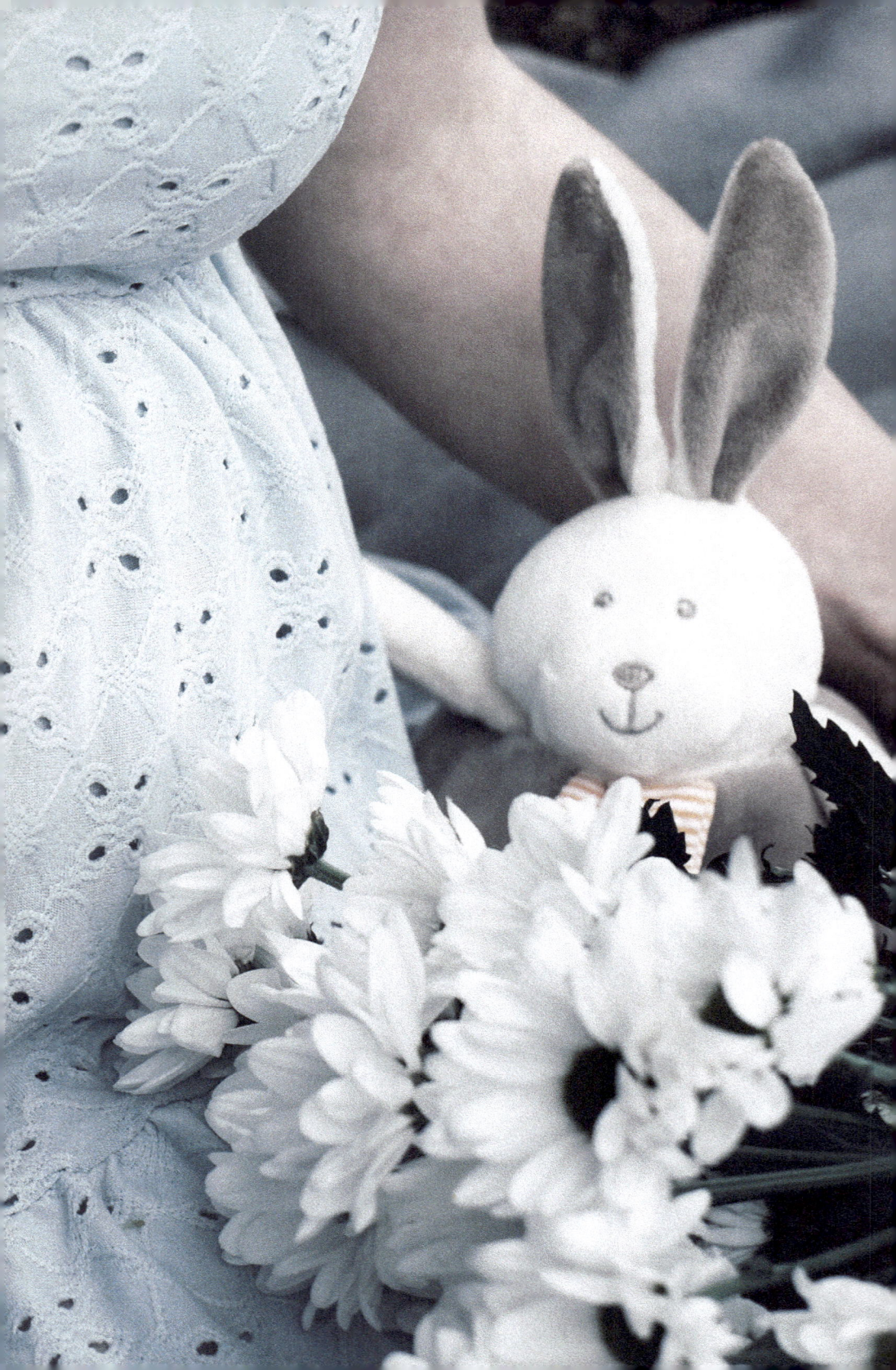

Chapter 21: Post Birth Changes for Mom

The first few days after birth, you and your baby are beginning to get to know each other.

Many baby books talk about mother and baby bonding instantly, mum feeling an immediate overwhelming love and affection so that all other emotions fade into insignificance beside what she feels for her child. Of course, some women feel this, gripped by a kind of passion just as some fathers do. Many women talk about how guilty they feel because the bonding they expected just after the birth didn't happen till a few days, weeks, months later. As with all things in life, we are all different, and some will bond instantly with their child, while others may take a little longer.

This is Olivia's memory:

«I recall the birth of my daughter lying in a hospital feeling strange. There was a little person in the nursery (we weren't allowed to have our babies on the ward). That was my baby. I kept touching my stomach, amazed at how flat it was. It all seemed surreal. I went all through the motions of looking after my baby in a kind of daze, then my milk came in on day three, and sitting there feeding her looking at her beautiful blue eyes, I fell in love.

Have a baby close to you as much as you can, both of you. The more you can hold on and cuddle your baby, the more confident you will become, and the baby loves close contact.

Get as much rest as you can in these early days when the baby sleeps. That's the time for you to sleep. I understand that many women feel they must "do it all," a perfect house, perfect baby. Some women have told me that they must clean everything before the midwife comes to call. The housework can wait at this time, or if you have family and friends close by, let them help with some cleaning and cooking for you while you spend time with your baby.

If you decide to breastfeed, your midwife can help you with any questions you may have or contact the National Childbirth Trust. They run breastfeeding classes and have a helpline you can call for assistance. The number is found in the back of this book.

Remember to eat plenty of fresh food and keep up your calorie intake if you are breastfeeding.

If you would like to drop, weight take your time, significantly if breastfeeding, a varied diet without too much fatty food will help you lose weight gradually while keeping up the milk production. Breastfeeding uses up lots of energy, and you may be hungrier than usual. If you are hungry, have a snack of a piece of cheese or beans on toast or a bowl of cereal.

Giving birth is a passionate and strenuous experience; it's called labor for a reason, and it can be hard work. Your hormones alter significantly in the first few days after birth, and some women do feel more emotional than others while these changes are happening.

If you have a baby in the hospital after the birth, you will be moved into the postnatal ward. Some mums love being in hospital with other mums and their new babies, while others do not. It can be difficult as the other babies may disturb your rest. One of my friends discharged herself early so that she could get home for a rest. Nowadays, the stay in the hospital is very short, and most mothers go home after a day, with some only staying a few hours after birth before going home. Discuss the postnatal care with your midwife. It is additionally a great opportunity for you to let her know your preferences, whether you want to stay for a day or leave as soon after the birth as you can so that the staff in the hospital are aware of your wishes.

Following the birth, you will lose blood and have a discharge from the vagina. The loss will be hefty first, and you will need super penetrable sanitary towels to deal with this. Ensure that you only use sanitary towels until after your post-natal check as tampons can cause infections in the early weeks after the birth. While breastfeeding, some women notice that the discharge is more massive.

If breastfeeding, you may not have another period for some weeks or months after the birth, remember you can still fall pregnant in this time. You can fall pregnant from 21 days after the baby is born. One of my friends thought that she was "safe" as her periods hadn't started after the birth of her Son in February, she fell pregnant straight away and gave birth to twins in the next November!

Your abdomen will seem quite squidgy after birth. It is partly because the muscles have stretched. By eating a balanced diet and exercising, you'll soon get your shape back.

Once you get home with your baby, the community midwife will pop in and visit you at home for a few days. She is there is help and advises you in looking after yourself as well as the baby.

Going home with your baby can be very exciting. The more you handle, cuddle your baby, the more your confidence will grow. Just after Joshua's birth, the midwife gave him to me, saying to my daughter, let's give him to Granny to dress. And I thought oh goodie Granny's coming! Then suddenly realized this was me. I took that tiny person into the next room and began to dress him and put his nappy. My first thought was, "I haven't done this for years. What do I do?"

The more you do with your partner, the more you will both enjoy the baby. Your partner may not be able to breastfeed, but he can help with bathing, changing nappies, dressing as well as cuddling. Many first-time dads are nervous about handling baby, be patient if he seems awkward at first, he'll soon get the hang of it.

You may need some help at first, not just with the chores, but to give you emotional support too. Many women want their partners with them at this time, and most employers now give some kind of paternity leave that gives you both some time to get to know your baby and begin the adjustment of having another person in your family. If you are a solo parent or your partner is unable to be with you, and you have no family close by, the National Childbirth Trust may be able to help you. They arrange various coffee mornings for new mums and have a "buddy system" whereby a new mum is befriended by someone who has already had a baby.

Look after yourself:

While you are feeding baby at night, finding time to rest in the day is essential. I know it's tempting to use baby's sleep time to catch up on chores, but this is the perfect time for you to rest too.

Some mums have said that at first, they feel awkward about taking a baby out. There are all those things to remember to take with you, but; taking a walk in the fresh air each day will be beneficial to both you and baby, and it will feel good to get out of the house.

With a new baby in the family, many relationships begin to change, your mother may not know what is expected of her, and she may try to do too much or not offer enough help for you. When Joshua was a baby, my daughter was living at home with us, and I was unsure of how much, if any, help she wanted. My husband and I kept out of her way as much as possible until we were asked to help her. When she had Logan, she and her partner were living in their own home, and I stayed away to give them time together and have just found out that she felt that I didn't give her enough help. Talk to the new grandparents and the rest of the family and let them know what you would like from them.

Crying – All baby's cry. It's their way of letting you know that they need something. They may be hungry, have wind or colic, feeling hot or cold, tired, lonely, and wanting company, or maybe they have a dirty nappy. If you have exhausted all of these and baby is still crying, hold him close and talk in a soothing voice. Movement, rocking gently helps. You will gradually recognize the meaning of the different cries that your baby gives and recognize when hungry, sleepy, etc.

The way that you feel is contagious. If you are upset, tense, frustrated, your baby will notice. For the past nine months, this tiny little person has been inside of you connected to your thoughts and emotions; when you felt happy, he felt happy. He knows your moods and feelings exactly. If when he is crying, you become tense when you pick him up. He will notice this and, in turn, may become tense in response to how you are feeling. Before you pick the baby up, remember your relaxation; take a deep breath, and begin to relax. Then once you are feeling calm, that is the time to pick him up.

The amount that babies sleep varies from baby to baby. Throughout the initial weeks,

some babies sleep for most of the time stuck between feeds, while others will be wide awake. As they develop older, they begin to create their routine of waking and sleeping, which changes as they grow. Each child is different; you will soon get used to your baby's routine.

When resting following the birth of baby, this is the ideal time to practice the relaxation techniques that you learned for birth. You can also continue using the CD to relax. Baby, too, may enjoy listing as this is familiar to him and will also relax him after the birth.»

Chapter 22: Baby Sleep Problems

At this age, you must accept a degree of disrupted sleep. It will pass, but my best advice is to give yourself a break. As I've said earlier, take all the help you are offered, don't give yourself a hard time about a messy house or a takeaway dinner, and know that it will soon be over, and everyone will be sleeping better. Just rest, enjoy your newborn, and recover from the birth and pregnancy. It's honestly not for long. There are a few sleep issues you may come up against that you may want to address for safety reasons or because they will make your life easier and aren't difficult to fix.

Not Being Able To Sleep On Their Back

At this age, it's recommended that babies are always put to bed on their backs, as any other position increases the risk of SIDS. One solution is to swaddle babies firmly in a blanket to help them feel secure and stop them from flailing. Another is to rock them gently to sleep, then move them into their bassinet or cot once they are deeply asleep. If you are consistent, she will eventually get used to sleeping on her back.

Not Knowing The Difference Between Night And Day

Babies have no sense of night or day and frequently wake throughout the night. We've looked at ways you can start to give them a sense of night and day, which will help over time. These include going outside and getting some natural light in the daytime and keeping nighttime waking as dark and quiet as possible, so she conveys that darkness is for sleeping.

Hunger

If you are breastfeeding, be sure to keep in touch with a lactation consultant to ensure that your baby is getting a good feed, as a hungry baby will find it hard to sleep. You may need to hold your baby or feed for a long time to get them off. Always get as much help as you need, and you can look forward to better sleep once the feeding routine is established.

With bottle-fed babies, again, ensure that the baby is getting enough food, checking the instructions for mixing the formula up carefully. A warm bath, followed by a feed, should provide a good sleep.

Two To Three-Month-Old Babies

Sleep Regression

Around this age, your baby should be sleeping better. However, you may also notice a sleep regression. It often accompanies a growth spurt or development leap and is characterized by an alert, active baby who shows no signs of wanting to sleep— setting your nighttime routine – bath, story, bed – so that your baby gets the message that nights are for sleeping, not playing. It will soon pass, but if you exhaust, see if you can get some extra rest or naps in the meantime.

Feeding through the night is another habit you can fall into, especially with breastfed babies. Your baby feeds little and often, leaving you exhausted. If you keep your baby in your room with you, you may be able to manage night feeds without fully waking up. But if you would like to stretch out the time between feeds, so you get more sleep, try, and give your baby a good feed last thing at night. Perhaps express a bottle of milk so your partner can take over one feed (although this may be more hassle than it's worth, and some breastfed babies will simply refuse a bottle and hold out for the breast.

Creating set times for bottles or breastfeeds in the daytime and trying to stick to them may also guide your baby towards a more regular sleeping and feeding pattern.

Teething Pain

Some babies may seem unsettled when they have a tooth coming through, with red cheeks and drooling. Extra cuddles, a teething ring, and a warm bath will all help to settle him. Teething will generally pass quickly, but if your baby seems to be incredibly unhappy, visiting your family doctor is worth a try. They may recommend some baby painkillers, which will help with sleep, too. Teething can also be used as a catch-all term for any delinquent behavior. Sometimes, it's worth looking a little deeper to discover any other solutions to delinquent behavior.

Four To Five-Month-Old Babies

Overstimulation

Around this age, your baby may drop a nap and start sleeping less in the daytime. It may lead to her being overtired at night and harder to settle. It's important to realize that an overtired baby may 'fire up' and become much more active, loud, and energetic than sleepy. It can be a sign of overstimulation, so if your baby seems overtired, try starting the bedtime routine a little earlier with all its associated sleep cues so they can catch up on sleep.

Sometimes, with an overtired baby, it takes longer for them to wind down, which can create a vicious circle of another late night followed by another unsettled day. It may help break the cycle' with a busy afternoon that includes some play and outside time, followed by a good feed, a long bath, and an early bedtime. No matter how alert your baby seems, keep in mind ideal sleep quantities for each age bracket and aim to get them – exhausted children won't learn and thrive as well as well-rested ones.

Six Months

Still Waking Up Wanting A Feed

Although we don't remember it in the morning, we all wake up during the night a couple of times and fall back to sleep again almost immediately with no memory of the event. Babies need to learn to fall back to sleep, preferably on their own without requiring too much help from their caregivers, past the age of about six months.

If you've been feeding your baby to sleep, you might now consider moving this feed to thirty minutes before bedtime and following it with a board book story and some lullabies in bed. You can expect some fussing at this change of routine, but if you are consistent, she will drift off without the bottle or breast if she is tired. Hopefully, this will make night-waking easier – if she learns that she can get back to sleep without a feed, just your voice and perhaps a gentle stroke should be enough to settle her again.

Of course, if you don't mind feeding through the night, don't feel you have to do this. But if you are exhausted during the day, it might be a good idea to introduce some gentle sleep training around six months to make day-to-day life more comfortable.

Early Waking

Some babies wake early, raring to go. You can try adjusting naps and bedtimes or put a black-out blind over the window to try and push her wake up time back a little. Another option is to bring her into your bed and hope that she drifts back to sleep.

Ultimately, though, early mornings are part and parcel of having a young baby, so getting to bed earlier yourself so you can handle the early start may be the best solution.

Healing Your Body Naturally

It's unbelievable that we can grow a small human and then produce enough food to nourish them during their early life. I am in awe every time I consider how amazing a woman's body is.

And breastfeeding does more than just nourish your baby. It reinforces the sacred bond between you and your child, encourages your uterus to resume its normal size, releases oxytocin, the love hormone, and can help you lose the extra weight essential to your healthy pregnancy.

But while breastfeeding is impressive, many moms struggle

with it. Breastfeeding can be painful, challenging, and just plain frustrating. But it doesn't have to be, and once you've persevered past the first couple of weeks, it gets a lot easier.

Difficulties with breastfeeding do not reflect negatively on your capabilities as a mother. Rather than allowing frustration and discouragement to build, I encourage you to seek help from a lactation consultant or midwife to help you troubleshoot. We aren't born with an innate understanding of breastfeeding. Because so much of our society has discouraged mothers from openly breastfeeding, we don't see it modeled as often as we should.

The World Health Organization advises exclusive breastfeeding for the first six months of life and then continued nursing until two years. Some women wean at a year, some women breastfeed longer than two years, and none of it is wrong. You'll discover what works for you and your child. And please remember, your nursing relationship is between you and your baby. Other people will have their views, but they are just opinions. They don't decide what is best for your baby—you do!

There will be many changes to your breasts, especially in the first 72 hours after birth. Your milk will turn up in, your breast will swell, and well, you may be uncomfortable. But not to worry! There are natural ways to find relief.

Here are a few tips to support you get breastfeeding more successful. If you feel like you need more support, get it! Don't hesitate to ask for help.

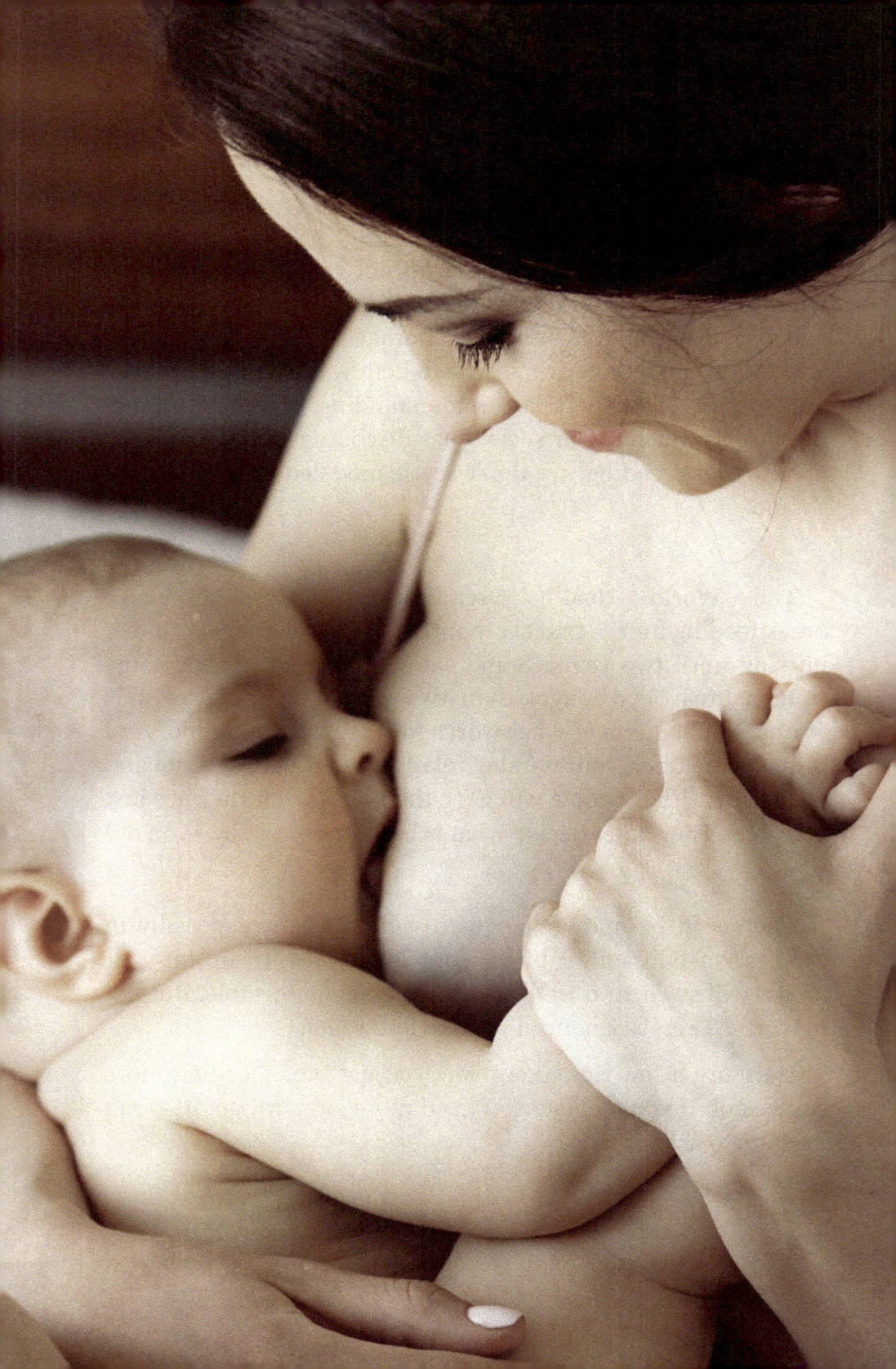

Chapter 23: Breastfeeding Basics: Tips for Successful Feedings

Get Comfortable. Find a chair that has back support and allows your feet to touch the ground. If your feet don't touch, get a stool to prop your feet on. It will help avert neck and back tension.

Use a Support Pillow. There are specialty breastfeeding pillows that offer support to babies, but you can use any pillows you choose. It will allow you and your baby some additional comfort.

Tummy-to-Tummy. Hold baby close and ensure both your bellies are making contact the entire time. Baby should be brought to you, not the other way around. It will reduce strain on your body and support a proper latch.

Baby's Alignment. Line the baby's ear, shoulder, and hip to make feeding and swallowing easier. The Baby's head should be tilted back just slightly. A chin-to-chest position makes a proper latch difficult.

Hamburger Hold. Wait. What? Grasp the breast, making your hand into a "C" shape so that the breast goes wide like a hamburger. Yes, there are better names out there, I'm sure, but hamburger is always how I held the visualization in my head.

Take Aim. Aim the nipple up towards the baby's nose so that when it is inserted, it is at the back of the baby's mouth, stimulating the palate.

Coax a Wide Open. Sometimes babe will only open partway. Avoid trying to place your nipple in a partially opened mouth—trust me, the pain will make you wish you didn't. Instead, rub your nipple across the baby's lip to encourage a wide open.

Chin Down, Tongue Down. Look for this position. Once the baby's mouth is open wide enough, and the tongue has dropped down, insert your nipple and the lower portion of the areola (the dark area around the nipple) into the baby's mouth.

Fish Lips. The top tip and bottom lip should fan out like a fish. If not, use your finger to open them up a bit more gently.

Baby's Latch: Baby Has an Important Role Too

A latch is essential for your comfort and the baby's success. Your baby's bottom lip should extend beyond the nipple onto the areola, the outer portion of the nipple that is generally darker. The nipple should angle up towards the back of the soft palate to the roof of the baby's mouth and the end. When the baby is nursing, make sure that you move the bottom lip to get around the areola.

If you are struggling with latch or pain every time you are

breastfeeding, meet with a lactation consultant. Sometimes some one-on-one guidance can make all the difference.

Signs of a Good Latch:

•Tongue is visible when the bottom lip is retracted.

•The jaw makes a circular motion, rather than a rapid chin movement.

•Chin touches breast.

•You hear swallowing instead of smacking noises.

•Ears wiggle and cheeks are rounded.

•Nipple does not appear flat when the baby is finished.

•Baby shows signs of satisfaction: hands open, falls asleep, falls off the breast, and seems relaxed.

Engorgement

"I remember when my milk came in. At first, the discomfort had me doubting if I should continue breastfeeding. My breasts were incredibly sore, but I realized my body was responding to my baby's needs, and honestly, breastfeeding was the only thing that brought me relief. It didn't take prolonged for us to find our rhythm, and when I remember wishing I could just stop breastfeeding. I laugh and am so thankful I didn't.

~Jennifer, mother of one

Within two to three days after giving birth, your body will begin producing breast milk and likely a lot of it. When your milk supply comes in, your breast will become engorged. Your body is trying to figure out how to meet the baby's demand, and its initial response is to bring in a lot of milk. It won't last forever—your body will, over time, get the supply and demand ratio down.

At the start, you and your baby establish a rhythm, which will help your body and brain understand what needs to happen. When the baby suckles, the breast is stimulated and signals your brain to release oxytocin. Your body then produces more milk. By feeding on demand (when the baby is hungry), your body will get a sense of what is needed.

Natural Remedies to Soothe Your Breasts

Cabbage Leaves. Cabbage leaves have been recommended by Midwives, Naturopathic Doctors, and mothers for ages. Place cabbage in your refrigerator (best bought before baby arrives) so that it is cold. Peel the outer leaf of the head of cabbage. Place one plate on the inside of each side of your bra to cover the breast completely. The cool cabbage leaf offers relief by increasing blood flow to the area, reducing inflammation, and allowing for easy milk flow.

It is also an excellent remedy for mastitis and blocked ducts (see Natural Remedies for Blocked Ducts).

Wear Comfortable Clothing. Underwire bras or clothes that feel too constricting can make your breasts feel worse. Some women feel better wearing a sports bra or no bra at all in the early days of breastfeeding. Equally uncomfortable is a bra or any clothing that is loose and brushes against the nipples, causing chaffing.

Sunlight and Fresh Air. Exposing your nipples to sunlight and fresh air for 20 minutes daily will reduce the growth of microbes and encourage the nipples to heal.

Feed Frequently. Allow baby to feed about every 2-3 hours in the beginning. Be sure to change breasts so that both are drained.

Hydrogel Pads. Easy-to-use cooling pads that soothe sore nipples.

Nipple Creams. Having a mouth on your nipple creates trauma to the skin and exposes your breast to a lot of moisture. It is not only uncomfortable but can leave you susceptible to infection. Applying barrier creams after every feeding can help soothe and protect your breasts.

First, dry the breast, and then apply calendula or another herbal salve to the nipple. Olive oil-based barrier creams tend to be well tolerated by infants and don't make them averse to feeding. Clean the nipple thoroughly before breastfeeding again.

Your skin is a significant barrier, and the first line of defense against microbial infections. If you lose that barrier or it's compromised through the microtrauma occurring from breastfeeding, then you're more susceptible to disease. Applying these barrier creams can help you protect yourself.

Calendula salve, which can easily be made at home or purchased, is excellent for healing the skin. Calendula is an antimicrobial herb that promotes tissue healing. It is perfect for sore, dry, cracked nipples and can also be used for diaper rash (bonus!).

See my homemade Calendula Salve Recipe:

Nourishing Calendula Salve

Calendula is a soothing, antimicrobial herb. This salve helps heal dry, cracked, or irritated tissue. I have used this salve for postpartum skin issues and my son's diaper rash with great success.

Ingredients:

- 8 ounces of calendula oil (make your own or purchase)
- 1-ounce beeswax
- 1 tablespoon vitamin E oil
- Glass jars 2 to 4 ounces

Directions:

Place herbs oil over a double boiler and gently warm. Slowly add beeswax until it melts. If you'd like a firmer salve, add more Beeswax and less for a softer balm. To test, dip a butter knife into the mixture, remove and allow to cool in the freezer.

Once you've achieved the desired consistency, remove from

the heat, and add vitamin E oil. Quickly pour into mason jars and allow to cool.

Store in a cold room. This salve will keep for about a year.

Yields 8 ounces of salve

What if my nipples are cracked and bleeding?

You may be able to heal your nipples naturally using nipple creams. However, if this issue persists, it may be a sign of improper latch. It wouldn't hurt to speak with a lactation consultant to see if there are any techniques you could employ to help yourself heal. You must tell your healthcare worker if you suspect infection—high fever, chills, body aches, red tissue, and foul-smelling discharge.

You can continue to breastfeed despite the bleeding. The blood will not hurt the baby.

Having a mouth always on the breast tissue with all of the moisture that brings can be very aggravating to the skin. If pain lasts more than 1-2 weeks or you're very concerned that something's wrong with your ability to breastfeed or produce milk, definitely meet with your healthcare practitioner.

Natural Remedies for Blocked Ducts

Blocked ducts are simply a backup of milk that can't be expressed. Sometimes it feels like a little Super Ball or maybe like a hard or a firm cord in the breast tissue. Inadequate breast emptying can be familiar with breast pumps. Still, it may also arise from being rushed, feeling stressed, going too long between feedings, compression on the breast, illness, or baby not feeding efficiently. Or maybe there's no good reason, and you've got a blocked duct. Whatever the reason, the remedy is to empty the breast.

If a blocked duct goes untreated, it can lead to mastitis, so it is best to act quickly.

Chapter 24: What Do I Need to take in the Hospital?

What goes in a hospital bag, and when should I get it ready? Regardless of whether you are having a home, hospital, or midwifery-unit birth, you need to pack a bag, so everything is in one place and the case of emergencies, at least two weeks before your due date. Your midwife will present you with a list tailored to your specific hospital/midwifery unit, but here are some things that you might want to include.

- Your birth plan if you have penned one.
- Medication/List of medication for any pre-existing conditions/illnesses you may have.
- Things to help you relax or pass the time (music, magazines).
- Loose and comfy clothing to wear during labor. Natural fibers are a better choice than human-made, as they let your body breathe more. You will probably need a few changes throughout labor, so make sure to pack about three sets. Some women may prefer to be naked throughout labor, but it is probably wise to fill them just in case. Don't forget to pack a comfortable outfit to wear home!
- About 24 extra-absorbent sanitary pads (Maternity ones with wings are a good idea).
- Sponge/cloth or a water-spray to help keep you cool during labor.

- Front-opening, or loose-fitting nighty or tops for breastfeeding; 2 or 3 supportive but comfortable bras (make sure to take nursing bras if you are breastfeeding).
- Breast pads.
- At least 5 or 6 pairs of pants.
- Toiletry Bag.
- Towels.
- Dressing gown and slippers
- Clothing (make sure you include a hat) and nappies for the baby.
- A shawl to wrap the baby in.
- A camera to capture those all-important first moments.

Think about getting to and from the hospital, and make sure you have a contingency plan, in case of unexpected problems with transport. Reason about the path you will take to allow for unforeseen holdups, e.g., roadworks. Remember, you can always call an ambulance!

NB: make sure you have a rear-facing car seat (and you disable any associated airbags). Please get expert advice, and ensure you know the new car seat regulations that come into effect on 1st March 2017.

If you are getting a home birth, you will need to discuss this with your midwife to ensure you have everything required. But at the very least, you will need clean linen and towels available for the midwife to use, sanitary pads, and clothing for when your baby arrives. You also ought to think about where you want to give birth and if you need to hire specialist equipment, e.g., a birthing pool.

Many people have mobile phones, but it can be handy to keep a written list of important contact details: Your hospital and midwife phone numbers; your partner/birth partner's phone number; your hospital reference number, as they will ask for this when you phone to say you are on your way.

Home Equipment Considerations

Babies require a lot of attention and come with a lot of baggage, literally! You may be thinking about where I start, as there are many items to buy before your baby is born. If this is your first baby, you may want to buy everything in sight, but just be aware you may find you don't need it all straight away. You will discover family and friends who will want to help let them!

Below is a list of items you may need immediately:
- Moses basket and stand
- Sheets and waffle blanket
- Changing table
- Baby monitor
- Baby bouncer
- Pram
- Breastfeeding pillow (if required)
- Sterilizer and bottles
- Baby formula (if bottle feeding)

- A baby baths
- Nappy bag
- Scented nappy sacs

Possible purchases are:
- Bottle warmer (a jug of hot water will suffice)
- Breast pump
- Nappy bucket (for terry nappies to be collected by an agency)
- Nappy Disposal Bin (these are specialist bins that lock odors away!)
- Dummies (if you think you want your baby to have one)

These things can wait to be purchased later:
- Cot
- Highchair
- Safety gate and catches
- Buggy

Newborns need a lot of attention. Make sure you gather a supply of necessary equipment a couple of weeks before your due date.

Some of the apparent items your baby will need are:
- Nappies (terry or disposable).
- Baby wipes.
- Baby powder,
- Nappy rash ointment/cream,
- Baby oil/lotion,
- Baby shampoo.

Less obvious items are:

- Nail scissors (specifically for newborns).
- Baby brush.
- Baby thermometer.
- Laundry powder that is hypoallergenic,
- Thermometer for your bathtub (many parents use the elbow in the water technique, satisfactorily), but whatever you use, be sure to put the cold water into the bath first, then the hot. This way, you avoid the possible risk of burns to the baby.

During the first weeks after your baby's arrival, you may not leave the house often to buy all the necessary items, so make sure you accept help when offered. Babies go through tons of nappies but do not overstock, as they change size frequently. If you chose not to breastfeed or cannot, you would need to buy formula milk.

NB: Do not makeup bottles with water straight from the tap. It needs to be freshly boiled and left to cool for no more than 30 minutes before making up the milk.

You will want to buy clothes for your baby, but please remember many people may gift you baby clothes. An item you might want to buy is a swaddle blanket. It keeps your baby warm and comfortable after being born.

Other items to buy include:

- Baby-grows/onesies.
- Socks.
- No-scratch mittens.

- Leggings,
- T-shirts,
- Cardigans/jumpers.
- Coats.
- Hats.
- Bibs.
- Burp cloths/muslins.

Remember that depending on when your baby is born, weather plays a factor when deciding which clothes to buy. Babies grow up fast, so there is no need to buy too many clothes before they are born.

It's not just your baby that needs things ready at home for, after the birth, you will too. Some items are Nursing bras, breast pads, sanitary pads, nipple cream, comfy clothing, a supply of nutritious snacks and foods. Yet again, if people offer to cook for you, take them up on the offer! You will more than likely be able to reciprocate one day.

Conclusion

After reading all of this, you are now feeling one of two ways. You are amazed that it is this simple and are ready to work on making birth easier for yourself, or you are in total disbelief that it can be this easy, and there must be more to it.

For those of you who don't believe it can be that easy, I suppose you have two choices. Do everything in the book anyway and hope for the best or do a little more research into this birth malarkey and find something that does convince you it works, because it does.

I authored this book to show you that birth can be different if you want it to be, so if it has even got you considering that there are ways to improve your chances of an easy birth, then my work here is done. It is now down to you to choose what to do with that idea.

Summary and a possible plan of action:

• Prepare your body by watching your posture, doing your pelvic floor exercises right, and trying perineal massage if it is something you want to do.

• Prepare your mind and your spirit

• Practice relaxing your body correctly and fully until you can do it yourself with no or little guidance.

• Ensure you have chosen a place to give birth where you can create a home-from-home style environment and pack things that will make you feel loved, safe, and secure in your hospital bag.

• Practice breathing in and out slowly, and with control, so you are ready to use the technique with the early contractions, even if they are short ones.

- Practice the massage techniques with your birth partner and remember that you can help your hormones along if you need to.

- Have a read over the different drugs again and make sure you know their side effects to make an informed choice when you are in labor. Practice the visualization techniques to use when you are finding things tough.

- Make sure you are familiar with the BRAIN acronym and how it can get information about the options available to you.

- Remember to breathe through the last stage of labor and avoid forceful pushing if you can.

- Decide what you want to happen with the cord and the placenta after the baby has been put on your chest or stomach for skin to skin.

Do not worry. I know you will be a great mother. You had been preparing enough. You are ready for the real one.

Thank you, and good luck!

Notes

Notes

www.ingramcontent.com/pod-product-compliance
Lightning Source LLC
Chambersburg PA
CBHW051542020426
42333CB00016B/2050